Springer Series on the Teaching of Nursing

2005   **Teaching Nursing Care of Chronic Illness: A Storied Approach to Whole Person Care,** *P. Minden, RN, PhD, APRN-BC, and C. Gullickson, RN, PhD, APRN, BC*

2004   **Research in Nursing and Health, 2nd edition: Understanding and Using Quantitative and Qualitative Methods,** *Carol Noll Hoskins, PhD, RN, FAAN, Carla Mariano, EdD, RN AHN-C, FAAIM, with contribs*

2004   **Developing An Online Course: Best Practices for Nurse Educators,** *Carol A. O'Neil, PhD, RN, Cheryl A. Fisher, MSN, RN, and Susan K. Newbold, RNBC, FAAN, MSN*

2004   **Academic Nursing Practice: Helping to Shape the Future of Healthcare,** *L. Evans, DNSc, FAAN, RN, and Norma M. Lang, PhD, FAAN, FRCN, RN*

2003   **Teaching Nursing in an Associate Degree Program,** *Rita G. Mertig, MS, RNC, CNS*

2001   **Educating Advanced Practice Nurses and Midwives: From Practice to Teaching,** *J. E. Thompson, RN, CNM, DrPH, FAAN, FACNM, R. M. Kershbaumer, MMS, RN, CNM, MSN, EdD, and M. A. Krisman-Scott, RN, PhD, FNP*

2000   **Nursing Informatics: Education for Practice,** *B. Carty, RN, EdD*

2000   **Distance Education in Nursing,** *J. M. Novotny, PhD, RN*

2000   **Community-Based Nursing Education: The Experiences of Eight Schools of Nursing,** *P. S. Matteson, PhD, RNC*

2000   **A Nuts-and-Bolts Approach to Teaching Nursing, 2nd ed.,** *V. Schoolcraft, RN, MSN, PhD, and J. N. Novotny, PhD, RN*

1999   **Clinical Teaching Strategies in Nursing,** *K. B. Gaberson, PhD, RN, and M. H. Oermann, PhD, RN, FAAN*

1999   **Integrating Community Service into Nursing Education: A Guide to Service-Learning,** *P. A. Bailey, EdD, RN, CS, D. R. Carpenter, EdD, RN, CS, and P. A. Harrington, EdD, RN, CS*

1999   **Teaching Nursing in the Era of Managed Care,** *B. S. Barnum, RN, PhD, FAAN*

1998   **Developing Research in Nursing and Health: Quantitative and Qualitative Methods,** *C. N. Hoskins, PhD, RN, FAAN*

1998   **Evaluation and Testing in Nursing Education,** *M. H. Oermann, PhD, RN, FAAN, and K. B. Gaberson, PhD, RN*

1996   **Using the Arts and Humanities to Teach Nursing: A Creative Approach,** *T. M. Valiga, RN, EdD, and E. R. Bruderle, MSN, RN*

1995   **Teaching Nursing in the Neighborhoods: The Northeastern University Model,** *P. S. Matteson, RNC, PhD*

1994   **The Nurse As Group Leader: Third Edition,** *C. C. Clark, EdD, RN, ARNP, FAAN*

1993   **A Down-to-Earth Approach to Being a Nurse Educator,** *V. Schoolcraft, RN, MS, PhD*

1993   **An Addictions Curriculum for Nurses and Other Helping Professionals: Vols. I and II,** *E. M. Burns, RN, PhD, FAAN, A. Thompson, RN, PhD, and J. K. Ciccone, MA, APR, Editors*

1991   **The Nurse Educator in Academia: Strategies for Success,** *T. M. Valiga, RN, EdD, and H. J. Streubert, RN, EdD*

The authors are nurse educators who each have extensive clinical experience, Dr. Gullickson in the medical-surgical arena and Dr. Minden in mental health. Dr. Gullickson is a geriatric nurse practitioner and Dr. Minden is certified as a psychiatric nurse clinical specialist. They share an interest in end-of-life care and both have completed the ELNEC faculty preparation course. In addition to their love of teaching, both have a passion for using humor as a therapeutic tool and have completed research relevant to this. They each have several publications on the topic and have presented at national and international conferences.

Pamela Minden, PhD, RN, APRN, BC
Associate Professor of Nursing
Edgewood College–Nursing Department

A Registered Nurse for twenty-seven years, Dr. Minden earned a bachelor's degree from Arizona State University, a master's degree in psychiatric/mental health nursing from Boston University, and a doctorate in curriculum and instruction from the University of Wisconsin–Madison. Prior to joining the Nursing Department at Edgewood College in 1993 she worked in a variety of clinical, consultative, and administrative capacities. A special interest in the spiritual dimension of health and alternative care approaches has led her to pursue advanced training in hypnosis, strategic family therapy, and parish nursing.

Colleen Gullickson, PhD, RN, APRN, BC
Professor of Nursing
Edgewood College–Nursing Department

A nurse educator for the last twenty-five years, Dr. Gullickson earned a bachelor's degree from the University of Wisconsin–Milwaukee, a master's degree in nursing from University of Wisconsin–Madison, and a doctorate in nursing from the University of Illinois–Chicago Medical Center. She completed post-masters work at Marquette University and is certified as a geriatric nurse practitioner. She taught at the University of Colorado–Denver and the University of Wisconsin–Madison before accepting a faculty position at Edgewood College in 1993.

Teaching Nursing Care
of Chronic Illness

Pamela Minden, RN, PhD, CS
Colleen Gullickson, RN, PhD, APNP, BC

 Springer Series on the
Teaching of Nursing

Springer Publishing Company, Inc.
11 West 42nd Street, 15th Floor
New York, NY 10036-8002

Acquisitions Editor: Ruth Chasek
Production Editor: Janice Stangel
Cover design by Joanne Honigman

04 05 06 07 08 / 5 4 3 2 1

Library of Congress Cataloging-in-Publication Data

Minden, Pamela.
    Teaching nursing care of chronic illness : a storied approach to whole person care / Pamela Minden, Colleen Gullickson.
        p. ; cm. — (Springer series on the teaching of nurisng
    Includes bibliographical references and index.
    ISBN 0-8261-2513-1 (alk. paper)
    1. Chronic disease—Nursing—Study and teaching. 2. Holistic nursing—Study and teaching. 3. Nursing—Study and teaching.
    [DNLM: 1. Education, Nursing. 2. Chronic Disease—nursing.
3. Curriculum. 4. Holistic Nursing—methods. WY 18 M663t 2005]
    I. Gullickson, Colleen. II. Title. III. Series: Springer series on the teaching of nursing (Unnumbered)
RT120.C45M56 2005
610.73'6'0711—dc22   2004023305

Printed in the United States of America by Integrated Book Technology.

We dedicate this text to the numerous students, clients, colleagues, and friends who shared their stories so others might learn what it means to live a life in the face of chronic illness. Their wisdom continues to humble and inspire us.

Contents

Preface		*vii*
1.	Living a Life With Chronic Illness	1
2.	Understanding Our Educational Environment	9
3.	Using Stories to Teach Whole-Person Care in Chronic Illness	21
4.	Teaching the Theory Component	43
5.	Teaching the Clinical Component	87
6.	Using the Experiences of Students	133
Appendix A. Case Examples		147
Appendix B. Sample Wellness Interviews		159
Appendix C. Sample Wellness Group Documentation		169
Appendix D. Clinical Evaluation Tools		185
Appendix E. Sample Completed Clinical Evaluation Tools		195
Appendix F. Adrian's Story		209
Appendix G. John's Story		223
Index		*241*

Preface

No doubt there are a variety of reasons for choosing to read this book. Perhaps you are new to nursing education and are looking for specific how-to information. Maybe the title piqued your interest because you wonder, "What is different about teaching chronic illness?" Whatever your motivation, we hope our storied approach to teaching whole-person care for individuals and families faced with chronic illness will encourage and inform both those in nursing practice and in nursing education.

We are nurse educators, and each of us has over 25 years of clinical experience, Colleen's experience is in the medical-surgical arena and Pamela's is in mental health. In addition to being doctoral-prepared teachers, Colleen is a geriatric nurse practitioner, and Pamela is certified as a psychiatric nurse clinical specialist. Our intent is to provide a comprehensive portrait of a theory course and a clinical course in chronic illness. Paired these courses serve as a conduit for teaching about the provision of nursing care with people experiencing enduring health concerns that impinge on the lives they want to lead. Both courses emphasize long-term management of complex physical and mental problems occurring at a variety of age levels, and the importance of multidisciplinary collaborative planning and continuity of care. Each takes into consideration not only the effects of disease and disability on the individual, but also on the individual's support system and on the larger community.

The courses are part of a 4-year baccalaureate nursing program at Edgewood College in Madison, Wisconsin. They are positioned in the middle of five semesters of nursing coursework that are each designed to reflect six curricular strands: caring, health, client/person, professional nursing, environment, and critical thinking. These strands, which are integral to each nursing course and the overall program, become increasingly complex at each level of the curriculum.

In their first nursing semester, students learn about community-based primary prevention across the lifespan, and in their next semester, they learn about secondary prevention with adults in acute-care settings. The chronic illness courses then expand the focus to tertiary prevention, move the definition of client from that of an individual or a family to groups, and place students in both inpatient and community settings to promote understanding of the need for a continuum of care.

Situating the chronic illness courses in the third semester of the nursing program allows students to develop confidence and competency in more familiar skills (e.g., communication, interviewing) and concrete skills (e.g., physical cares, IVs, medications) before exposing them to the complex and controversial issues surrounding chronic illness management. In these two courses, they observe firsthand the dynamic interdependence between individuals with chronic illnesses, their immediate supports, and the more global health care system. The two courses are crucial in preparing students to care for families with complex health concerns in the fourth semester and with communities at risk in their final semester. In essence, the chronic illness courses move the students from a myopic perspective to a more panoramic one.

Chapter 1 identifies the impetus for developing and teaching courses in chronic illness at Edgewood College. It then briefly explores how the hegemony of the biomedical model and the character of chronic illness conspire to create negative mindsets in our students when they first venture into tertiary care.

A context for understanding how we teach about chronic illness is provided in Chapter 2, where you will find a brief overview of the history and mission of the academic institution where we have taught for the last 11 years. We reflect there as well on how the values of justice, truth, compassion, community, and partnership inform and guide the liberal arts curriculum that forms the foundation for nursing education at our college. The chapter delineates key aspects of Edgewood's nursing curriculum, where the two chronic-illness courses are pivotally positioned in the latter part of the junior year.

The theoretical frame in which the two courses are embedded is presented in Chapter 3. Our storied approach to whole-person care, a pedagogical integration of two cognitive modes—the logico-scientific and the narrative—is also discussed. Three organizing themes—self-regulation, stigma, and caregiver issues that serve as lenses for learning the clinical knowledge and skills necessary for providing holistic care to individuals and families encountering challenges associated with chronic illness—are then elaborated on and illustrated.

At the inception of the chronic illness courses in 1996, Edgewood nursing faulty as a whole collaborated to create specific learning objectives for each, which continue to direct curriculum development and assessment of student learning. These are delineated in chapters 4 and 5 respectively, as are our methods for achieving them. Chapter 4 centers on what and how we teach in the theory course. Classroom strategies to promote understanding of the lived experience of chronic illness, and the knowledge and skills to manage it are elucidated. Chapter 5 explains our instruction methods in both the psychosocial/spiritual and medical/surgical components of the clinical course, where students learn to shift their focus of care from "doing to" to "being with."

Chapter 6 brings us metaphorically full circle as three students who return to our classroom as guest speakers recount parts of their learning journeys. Though unsolicited, their affirmation of our teaching reassures that our methods can transform skepticism about chronic care into a powerful appreciation for the courage and creativity of persons living a life under the perpetual influence of illness. Their comments illuminate the student side of the teaching-learning process and exemplify the fact that, as educators, we will never know how our students are internalizing our course content unless we ask.

Regardless of how or why you have acquired this text, we trust you will find it amply supplied with scholarly and practical information for enhancing clinical and classroom instruction, especially as relates to the care and management of long-term health concerns. We hope as well that it inspires nursing practitioners, educators, and students to reach outside their comfort zones, as have we and our students, to promote the clients we have been privileged to serve, quality whole-person care. We are grateful for all they have taught us and for their opportunity to pass it along to you.

Living a Life With Chronic Illness

In 1900, the average life expectancy for an American was 50 years, and the death rate was 1,720 per 100,000. A high incidence of disease that was largely communicable and for which there was but limited treatment meant illness and dying trajectories were relatively short. The focus of health care was thus necessarily on comfort (End-of-Life Nursing Education Consortium, 2001, p. m22).

The biomedical model, variously called the clinical or disease model, is the most prevalent framework for understanding health and illness in contemporary Western culture. Often credited with enhancing the quantity and quality of human life by advancing treatment of infectious disease and acute bodily trauma, its efficacy is apparent in the fact that, by 1997, the average life expectancy in the United States had increased to 76 years, and the death rate had dropped to 865 per 100,000. Notwithstanding its obvious utility, assumptions inherent in the biomedical model can lead to a precariously narrow view of humans and health. Conceptualization of a person as a biochemical system whose whole can be inferred from its parts, acceptance of the Cartesian mind/body dichotomy, and a perception of health and illness as opposing poles on a linear continuum conspire to obscure the interactive role social, mental, cultural, political, economic, environmental, and spiritual factors play in health.

The reductionism characteristic of the Western world for the past 300 years is apparent in the distinct disciplines and subjects that order knowledge, the analytic techniques developed that focus on discrete factors, and even in the way we are taught to perceive different parts of ourselves (Wheatley, 1999, p. 29). Over 25 years ago, *Clinical Nursing: Pathophysiological & Psychosocial Approaches*, a book described as "The most comprehensive and authoritative text available in professional clinical nursing" (Beland & Passos, 1975, book jacket), advocated the synthesis and integration of biological, social, cultural, and behavioral knowledge, rather than simply viewing the patient from a strict biomedical model. Out of print for over a decade, this widely acclaimed book reasserted an expectation promulgated by Nightingale that nursing practice should take into consideration more than physical-care needs. The emergence of nursing diagnosis in the early 70s helped set the stage for this restoration, in part by providing a vocabulary to describe what nursing is and does. Nursing diagnoses delineate the discipline's phenomenon of concern—that is, human responses to actual and potential health threats. Nurses treat those human responses.

Like medicine, nursing seeks to help people reach, retain, and regain health, though an orientation toward cure guides the former discipline, and care is a more primary compass for the later. Paradoxically, *progress* measured as increased longevity and attributed to the biomedical model is accompanied by an increased incidence of chronic illness.

Nearly 50% of the 276 million Americans in the year 2000 had some type of chronic condition (Partnership for Solutions, 2003). Close to 60 million Americans now suffer from multiple chronic conditions, with 3 million of these having as many as 5 (Partnership for Solutions, 2003). Chronic medical conditions ranging from paralysis, Alzheimer's disease, mental disorders, and HIV/AIDS to allergies, asthma, diabetes, and high blood pressure affect men, women, and children of all ages, ethnicities, and income levels and are the leading reason why people seek medical attention (Anderson, 2003). Yet, national surveys of 1,238 physicians, 1,663 Americans, and a convenience sample of 155 policy makers reflect a prevalent attitude that the current health care system is not adequately addressing the needs of those so afflicted (Anderson, 2003). Rantz, Marek, and Zwygart-Stauffacher suggest that due to "the stark realities of the sheer numbers of aging persons in our society, their increased risk of chronic illness, their economic power, and their demands as consumers," the future financial survival of health care organizations is closely linked to providing effective and efficient care for this population (p. 51).

Many people with chronic conditions require assistance from family caregivers and a variety of professional providers. Promoting health in the occurrence of chronic illness requires the efforts of a collaborative multidisciplinary team providing a continuum of care extending way beyond the confines of today's restricted hospital stays. Intervening effectively necessitates exceeding biomedical obsession with physical integrity and helping afflicted individuals to manage their symptoms, obtain relief from suffering, cope with their related fears, and maintain their highest level of functioning. It necessitates attention to spiritual concerns, as well as the psychosocial and bodily needs that Beland and Passos insisted nursing address. Providing care in the occurrence of chronic illness entails venturing beyond neat and tidy, but false dichotomies in contemporary nursing texts still exist and are apparent in common binaries like mind and body, health and illness, or acute and chronic. It necessitates being alert to a proclivity toward medicalization, which allows thoughts, feelings, and behaviors that depart from accepted norms to be diagnosed and treated as disease. In other words, it requires thinking and acting holistically.

With care as its foundation, nursing would seem ideally suited to meet the above noted requirements, but long-standing hegemony of the biomedical model has led many nurses to reflexively find acute-care settings preferable. Though it would be very hard at any point in time to find a nurse who saw only the physical aspects of care as relevant, opportunities to identify and cure pathology often seem more attractive than helping one cope with its irreversible ravages. The January 2002 issue of the *American Journal of Nursing* includes an editorial that asks, "Is nursing adequately addressing the needs of the chronically ill?" (Mason, Leeman, & Funk, 2000, p. 7). The authors posit that lack of time in the primary-care setting, coupled with care-delivery models focused on acute care and cure, hinder the health care system's ability to meet the needs of the chronically ill. A primary contention is that current and future nursing research studying the lives of individuals with chronic illness will help clinicians "identify ways to better support patients in their efforts to live with illness" (Mason, Leeman, & Funk, 2000, p. 7). To promote that inquiry, the *American Journal of Nursing* publishes a quarterly column entitled "Living with Illness."

Clearly, Nursing, as represented in the journal of its professional organization, recognizes the vast need for better information and teaching about caring for individuals living with chronic illness. Ironically, however, the title of the editorial calling our attention to this need underscores a common propensity to define the individual with a chronic illness as the illness. In other words, *the chronically ill* takes the tenor of a proper noun, inadvertently implying all who occupy the category are the same. In our experience, that perceived uniformity is often cast with a negative patina.

Few students come to the courses described in this book excited about doing *chronic care,* and even fewer look forward to the possibility of doing it with *the mentally ill, the elderly, or the persistently infirmed and/ or dying.* In general, students come to us with a plethora of negative stereotypes and a desire to just get through the courses as quickly as possible. They would prefer to continue in acute care settings, where they can learn to use the most current and sophisticated equipment so they can "fix" people or "make them better" and send them home.

In summary, the ever-escalating incidence and prevalence of chronic illness, coupled with a current shortage of nurses interested in and prepared to meet the complex needs of those experiencing it, motivated the development of Edgewood's theory and clinical courses in chronic illness. Our goal in teaching them is to create a learning environment that fosters in our students the interest, curiosity, and empathy necessary for providing compassionate, whole-person care, especially when the need for care is ambiguous, amorphous, and/or all encompassing.

CHRONIC ILLNESS—A LACK OF ALLURE

Described variously, chronic illness commonly is regarded as progressive and deteriorating in nature and without the possibility of complete cure or prevention. Miller and Dzurec (1993) note that empiricist researchers name variables of interest before studying them so that they *can* study them. They " . . . expect that the chosen name is, indeed, what it says it is, even more appropriately, what the literature says it is" (p. 17). It is beyond the scope of this text to elaborate the various nuances of hanging a label on this particular phenomenon. The interested reader will likely find Lubkin and Larsen (2002, chapter 1) useful in that regard. Curtain's and Lubkin's 1995 definition of chronic illness as "the irreversible presence, accumulation, or latency of disease states or impairments that involve the total human environment for supportive care and self-care, maintenance of function, and prevention of further disability" cited there (p. 8) provides one reasonable starting point for exploration of what this complex concept means for nursing practice.

Throne and Paterson (1998) note that in the last two decades, conceptualizations of individuals diagnosed with chronic illness have shifted "from a focus on loss and burden toward images of health within illness, transformation, and normality" (p. 173). Correspondingly representation of such individuals in the professional literature has gone from that of passive recipients of professional health care to active partners and competent decision makers; in other words, "from patient to partner" (Throne & Paterson, p. 176). Preoccupation with loss and suffering or with the potential for growth and transformation associated with chronic illness obscures what is not so much a state of being (e.g., being disabled) as a process of continual change and adaptation. To preclude our students from drawing simplistic conclusions about what is actually a multifaceted occurrence, we purposely do not provide them with definitive definitions of chronic illness. Rather, we invite them to explore with us the meaning of chronic illness from a variety of perspectives, including their own and those derived from personal experience with family, friends, and clients encountered in earlier courses. We seek not so much to develop a discrete grasp of what chronic illness is as to discern its significance for real people encountering its challenges and rewards as they go on living or prepare for death. Charmaz's (1991) seminal study of the significance of chronic illness from the perspective of those who have experienced it titled, *Good Days, Bad Days*, has proven to be one of the most pliant springboards for launching our students into such exploration.

Chronic illness affects the self to a greater or lesser degree depending on the extent to which it impinges on various aspects of the person's everyday life (e.g., time, work, leisure, relationships), the social context in which the person exists, and how the individual defines the illness (Charmaz, p. 7). Charmaz notes that "people experience serious chronic illness in three ways: as an interruption of their lives, as an intrusive illness, and as immersion in illness" (p. 9). When chronic illness is perceived as an interruption, the person first looks for complete or near-complete recovery and later hopes to regain the last plateau of wellness (p. 13). With intrusion, the chronic illness becomes a permanent part of life that demands continued attention and allotment of time, and it forces accommodation (p. 42). At the point of immersion, the illness is no longer simply added to the structure of one's life; rather, life is reconstructed upon illness (p. 76). The journey from interruption to immersion generally proceeds over alternatively rough and more even byways (p. 9). "Certainly medical treatment can alter how someone experiences a chronic illness. Technical advances may permit keeping an intrusive illness in the background of life. Conversely, iatrogenic effects can bring it into the foreground" (p. 10).

Contemporary views of chronic illness and on those afflicted with it clearly depart from current images of people facing acute illness (Throne & Paterson, 1998, p. 176). Students arrive in our nursing care in chronic illness courses fresh from a semester devoted principally to secondary prevention and to the care of adults experiencing episodic disruptions in health. Though there they were introduced to health "as a dynamic, perpetual, and multifaceted process that is subjectively experienced, sometimes objectively manifested, and has implications for the physical, mental, social and spiritual functioning of individuals, specific aggregates, entire societies, and the universe as a whole" (Minden, 1999) many students still enter the chronic care courses fixated on health indicators that are observable or measurable.

Seven earlier class periods highlighted psychosocial and spiritual concerns such as pain, stress, crisis, anxiety, grief, therapeutic boundaries, and group and milieu treatment. Nonetheless, initial attempts to engage students in our chronic care courses in the holistic thinking necessary for intervening in the series of inevitable ups and downs challenging how one can live one's life are often frustrated by the students' fascination with physiological care operationalized as starting IVs and engaging in other technical skills supposed to be indicative of "real nursing." A developmental predilection toward believing that there are right answers for every clinical question that they will master if they can just figure out what it is their instructors want initially obscures any potential passion for understanding and interceding in chronic illness that we hope to foster.

Like persons experiencing chronic illness as interruption, students come to our courses assuming illness is a temporary phenomenon and that with time and the "right" care everything will return to "normal." They have little grasp of the limits of the technical skills they have been learning and the biomedical model from which these skills derive. It stands to reason that early in the experience of chronic illness clients expect biologically focused medical treatments often employed in acute illness to resolve their concerns and for students unaccustomed to treating chronic illness to share this misconception.

REFERENCES

Anderson, G. F. (2003). *Archives of Internal Medicine, 163*(4), 437–442. Available on line at *http://www.partnershipforsolutions.org/DMS/files/PPP_Paper.pdf*

Beland, I. L., & Passos, J. Y. (1975). (3rd Ed.). *Clinical Nursing: Pathophysiological & Psychosocial Approaches.* MacMillian Press.

Charmez, K. (1991). *Good days, bad days.* New Brunswick, NJ: Rutgers University Press.

End-of-Life Nursing Education Consortium. (2001). *Faculty guide.* Pomona, CA: American Association of Colleges of Nursing, City of Hope, and the Robert Wood Johnson Foundation.

Lubkin, I. M., & Larsen, P. D. (Eds.). (2002, 5th Ed.). *Chronic illness. Impact and interventions.* Boston: Jones and Bartlett Publishers.

Mason, D. J., Leeman, J., & Funk, S. G. (2002). Living with illness. *American Journal of Nursing, 102*(2), 7.

Miller, M. E., & Dzurec, L. C. (1993). The power of the name. *Advances in Nursing Science, 15*(3), 15–22.

Partnership for Solutions. (2003). Available on line at *http://www.partnershipforsolutions. org/statistics/prevalence.cfm*. Retrieved 6/17/03. A Partnership of John Hopkins University and the Robert Wood Johnson Foundation.

Rantz, M. J., Marek, K. D., & Zwygart-Stauffacher, M. (2000). The future of long-term care for the chronically ill. *Nursing Administration Quarterly, 25*(1), 51–58.

Throne, S., & Paterson, B. (1998). Shifting images of chronic illness. *Image: Journal of Nursing Scholarship, (30)*2, 173–178.

Wheatley, M. J. (1999). *Leadership and the new science*. San Francisco: Berrett-Koehler.

2

Understanding Our Educational Environment

I n this chapter, we step back to give you a synopsis of the educational context for teaching our students about nursing care in chronic illness. Familiarity with our academic setting is vital in that it is within the Edgewood College milieu that we shape our nursing curriculum. This text focuses on whole person care, emphasizing the importance of living a life in the presence of chronic illness. As you will discover in your reading, context is central in understanding the individuals we care for and learn from. Here we introduce you to Edgewood College, our nursing curriculum, and two important individuals who help us teach our chronic illness courses.

OVERVIEW OF EDGEWOOD COLLEGE

As an institution of higher education, Edgewood College is sponsored by the Sinsinawa Dominicans, a Congregation of Catholic nuns established in 1847 following Dominican traditions. The Congregation founded Edgewood College in 1927, initially as a junior college for women.

In 2003, we celebrated Edgewood's 75th anniversary and the 25th anniversary of our nursing program. Today, our college supports a total undergraduate and graduate enrollment of 2400 students, offering over 45 undergraduate majors in liberal arts and professional studies. In addition, Edgewood College offers graduate degrees in nursing, business administration, education, marriage and family therapy, and religious studies. The master of science degree in nursing encompasses three different concentrations: nursing administration, nursing education, and nursing as a health ministry.

The College's mission statement provides the foundation for all educational offerings and includes the following statement of values: "We foster open, caring, thoughtful engagement with one another and an enduring commitment to service, all in an educational community that seeks truth, compassion, justice, and partnership" (Edgewood College Undergraduate Catalogue, p. 10). Central to understanding educational mission statements and their role in guiding curricula is acknowledging that all education is values based. Regardless of the locale, institutional values direct the process and the outcome. What differs among settings is whether these values are implicit or explicit in their institutional expression.

VALUES

At Edgewood, the values of truth, justice, compassion, partnership, and community serve as the nucleus for our educational offerings. Understanding the intent and purpose of these is vital for faculty and staff as we strive to educate students as lifelong learners and responsible citizens in the global community. The five values are interconnected, with each requiring components of the others before any one can be realized. Each value is a process—an action oriented verb, something that is continuously ongoing rather than a static, definitive object. We believe they are universal and have relevance in any academic setting. Their significance for our nursing program and the chronic illness courses we teach is described in detail in the sections that follow.

Truth

Anyone's first uninformed response to hearing this value could easily be one of skepticism. Truth seems like an extremely omnipotent value, but whose "truth" are we referring to? In an article entitled, "The Value of Truth," Edgewood philosophy professor John Fields relates that

> Some, familiar with the role Dominicans played in the Inquisition, mistakenly think our call is to defend the truth, but it's really to be persistent in our efforts to perceive it. The emphasis is on the search. If we should become smug or complacent imagining we've once and for all captured the truth in dogmatic formulae, we've missed the point (Ashe, 2000, p. 2).

Expressed in other words, truth seeking becomes the "relentless search for ever-better ways to understand/express the vast array of human experience" (Leonard, as cited by Fields, 2003, p. 5). Critical to understanding the value truth is the inclusion of dialogue—truth speaking. Recognizing and respecting the potential multiplicity of other perspectives involves listening to what others have to say and bringing all voices into dialogue.

As Pamela notes in later chapters, "Any way of seeing is also a way of not seeing." Challenging our nursing students to acknowledge and respect other perspectives and bring these into the dialogic process is part of recognizing the value of truth. Remembering that truth, as a goal, may not be best represented by the current state, students are reminded that it's always possible that we have gotten it totally wrong.

Students in our chronic illness courses are exposed to the logico-scientific mode of inquiry as well as narrative mode as frameworks for truth seeking. Both frameworks present different perspectives on truth, yet both frameworks are equally compelling. By implementing educational strategies that endorse the relevance of both frameworks, we authenticate the value of truth seeking.

Justice

Justice involves behavior that recognizes the rights and responsibilities of all. Attorney Ray Eby-Booth, a 1992 Edgewood graduate, recognizes that the "hardest work of justice is understanding" (2003, p. 62). "While I learned a great deal about literature, education and art while I was at Edgewood—knowledge I will always take with me—the lesson that I lean on most every day is this: hard work to understand the facts and a willingness to be open to new ideas leads to understanding. Understanding applied equals justice in action" (p. 62).

Eby-Booth's insights have great relevance for our nursing students as their clinical courses expose them to vulnerable populations that all too readily fall through the cracks of the U.S. health care system. Whether working with the frail elderly or people who are uninsured or underinsured, who have often misunderstood or stigmatized conditions, or whose status as natives or refugees has jeopardized access to and quality of care, our nursing students learn about social (in)justice. They learn as well about individual and professional responsibility as they care for many clients who are ineligible to receive assistance from other sources but still require nursing services.

Compassion

Nursing literature is sated with information pertaining to caring. After all, aren't compassion and caring synonymous with nursing? What could we offer that is new or different from Nursing's ostensibly well-informed conceptualization? Dominicans view compassion as "mercy and empathy with another's suffering," and one of our colleagues, Professor Bob Reif, offers a simplification that resonates with nursing practice: "Compassion is the capacity to care for other people and for other living things" (Reif, 2003, p. 43).

Pamela describes this process as recognizing our shared humanity. Acknowledging intrinsic dignity and interdependence is an extremely important component in developing compassion and one that nursing literature often underemphasizes.

A second question is one of whether compassion can be taught. In reference to our clinical course, Pamela recognizes that "they (nursing students) didn't need me to teach them about compassion, they just needed an opportunity for expressing their innate capacity for it" (Minden, 2003, p. 41).

Partnership

Editorial news writer Neil Heinen (2003) suggests that although "we like to think of ourselves as rugged individualists, descendents of pioneers, forging our place in the world dependent on nothing but our wits," we ultimately seek partnerships.

In part because of the need for meaningful clinical placements, the success of the nursing department hinges on open, thoughtful engagement with a variety of individuals, programs, and organizations. Toward this end, we have made a commitment to place nursing faculty, not just preceptors, with our nursing students at every clinical site utilized. This simultaneously conveys an important message about our commitment to student learning and acknowledges and respects the present-day demands on nursing staff.

Sustaining our partnerships requires that they be mutually beneficial, with each partner receiving as much as they give. Staffing shortages, increased acuity, and limited resources can inhibit staff receptivity to students, who, without adequate supervision, can place an additional burden on a nursing unit or department. A strong faculty presence in our clinical courses helps bridge the gap between education and practice and sets the stage for collaboration, professionalism, and learning for all.

Recognizing the value of 'other' perspectives is fundamental to developing and sustaining partnerships. "Partnerships are relational and democratic. They are about seeing that no one is left out. They are about improving the life we live in common, in community" (Heinen, 2003).

Community

Two of Edgewood's staff express how the values of community and truth interact.

> Truths reached in solitary study are limited. It is only in community, in conversation with others, that ideas get challenged and enlarged, stretched and more clearly formed. Community also affirms creative ideas that are seeded in solitude. As study moves individuals to solitude, it also leads them back to community where dialogue can happen (Hopkins & Naughton, 2003, p. 18).

The learning community called Edgewood College is geographically located near the center of Madison, Wisconsin. As the state capital with a population of approximately 208,000 and home to the University of Wisconsin and its 40-some thousand students, the city presents a variety of opportunities and challenges for its residents. Sited on 55 acres next to a small lake, Edgewood College shares its campus with an elementary school and a high school, also under the sponsorship of the Sinsinawa Dominicans. This, coupled with the fact that Edgewood College is home to annual Elder Hostel educational events creates a unique "womb to tomb" learning community. Our communal campus and surrounding city affords the nursing program exceptional access to clients of various ages, backgrounds, and experiences.

As educators, we challenge our students to examine critically the communities in which they live, work, and interact, and to question who is included or not, who has voice, and who is silent and why. We want them to create connections beyond the walls of our college or their usual groupings that cultivate respect for all and encourage a shared search for truth. To facilitate this, we have developed a community-based nursing curriculum that recognizes the importance of a continuum of health activities and services for whole-person care. All of our clinical courses except one in the second semester when learning occurs principally in a nursing lab and on hospital units, include a community component such as outpatient clinics, social service agencies, neighborhood schools and centers, and client homes.

THE NURSING PROGRAM

Edgewood College's Dominican heritage sets a tone for service learning that is apparent in many of its undergraduate and graduate offerings. Clearly, service plays a major role in professional nursing, and knowing the clients we serve as nurses is vital. Our nursing program takes an inductive approach to teaching students about those who will be the focus of their concern, first introducing the care of the individual, then proceeding to families and groups, and ultimately to population aggregates. A progression from the most simple to the more complex is also apparent in the way the six curricular strands or themes of caring, critical thinking, health, client, environment, and professional nursing (noted in the Preface) are presented to students. The nursing courses are laid out so that those and other relevant concepts continually evolve as students move through the curriculum.

Progressive Strands and Program Objectives

The curricular strands, which are reflected in increasingly sophisticated ways at each level of the five semesters of the nursing program, guide the development of specific student outcomes for all clinical and theory courses. Agreed upon in advance by the faculty as a whole, these in turn serve as springboards for achievement of the following interdependent program objectives approved by the Wisconsin Board of Nursing as well as by Edgewood's Nursing Department. These six strands follow.

Caring: Establish therapeutic relationships with clients that demonstrate caring.

Health: Demonstrate critical thinking skills and caring practices to promote, maintain, and restore health.

Critical Thinking: Synthesize knowledge from nursing theory, research and practice; the humanities; and the natural and behavioral sciences to provide a basis for professional nursing practice.

Environment: Respond to environmental factors that influence the health of individuals, families, and communities.

Clients/Person: Collaborate with clients and colleagues in the process of identifying and organizing resources for the effective provision of health care.

Professional Nursing: Demonstrate professional behaviors that reflect accountability and commitment in nursing practice.

Program Requirements

Edgewood's Nursing Department admits 35–38 undergraduate students twice a year (spring and fall semesters) into its program, for a total undergraduate enrollment of approximately 150–170 students. The nursing major is comprised of a mixture of liberal arts and professional studies and qualified students usually begin nursing coursework in the second semester of their sophomore year.

Students earn 49 nursing credits in addition to 79 liberal arts credits for a total of 128 credits for graduation. Forty-nine nursing credits may appear low in contrast to other programs. However, courses that support the nursing major such as pathophysiology or microbiology are not counted as nursing credits. Only those courses taught by nursing faculty are regarded as nursing credits.

Presently, we are fortunate that our program is able to accommodate clinical placements for all students in mental health, maternal/child, and pediatrics, as well as the more standard medical-surgical and community health placements. Student experiences include 16 weeks of psychiatric/mental health nursing and 8 weeks of both pediatric and maternal/child nursing. The nursing courses and curricular strands are summarized in Table 2.1, where numbers ending in zero indicate theory courses and those ending in one indicate clinical courses.

VALUES APPLIED: PUTTING A FACE ON CHRONIC ILLNESS

The values elaborated earlier are one mark of an Edgewood College education and are apposite to the six curricular strands integrated throughout our nursing program. Together they form the principal

TABLE 2.1 Concept Development Throughout the Curriculum

Program Sequence	Semester 1	Semester 2	Semester 3	Semester 4	Semester 5
Courses →	**NRS 210:** Foundations of Professional Nursing **NRS 211:** Nursing Assessment and Intervention	**NRS 310:** Professional Nursing—Adult Health **NRS 311:** Caring—Adult Health Nursing	**NRS 340:** Professional Nursing—Long-Term Health Issues **NRS 341:** Collaborative Practice in Chronic Illness Management **NRS 390:** Research in Professional Nursing	**NRS 410:** Professional Nursing—Families in Transition **NRS 411:** Caring—Families in Transition **NRS 412:** Leadership Within the Health Care System	**NRS 460:** Professional Nursing Community Health **NRS 461:** Nursing Care With Aggregates **NRS 440:** Adult Health—Advanced Concepts in Acute Care
Concept →					
Health	Primary	Secondary	Secondary & Tertiary	Primary, Secondary & Tertiary	Primary, Secondary & Tertiary
Client	Individuals	Individuals	Individuals, Families and Groups	Families & Aggregates	Aggregates & Communities
Environment	Immediate Environment	Health Care & Changing Environment	Resource Allocation	Socio-political & Social Justice	Cultural Pluralism
	Safety	Safety	Safety	Safety	Safety

TABLE 2.1 (*continued*)

Program Sequence	Semester 1	Semester 2	Semester 3	Semester 4	Semester 5
Professionalism	Self, Clients, Peers, Professionals	Professional Issues & Organizations	Professional Issues & Organizations	Society	Society
	Image	Image	Image	Image	Image
Critical Thinking	Assessment & Planning	Assess, Plan, Implement & Evaluate using appropriate criteria	Assess, Plan, Implement & Evaluate using appropriate criteria	Contextual knowledge & Reasoned judgments	Contextual knowledge & Reasoned judgments
Caring	Viewing self and others as having intrinsic worth	Appreciates individuality	Appreciates individuality	Social responsibility	Social responsibility
		Maintains self esteem	Maintains self esteem	Advocacy	Advocacy
	Self empowerment	Empowerment of self and others	Empowerment of self and others		

underpinnings for preparing our graduates for moral leadership in the nursing profession and society. Simply described, they might appear rather flat, lifeless, or of little value. It is only in the context of human experience that these values have significance.

The courses detailed in this text are designed to teach nursing students about what it means to live a life with chronic illness so that they can ultimately provide competent, compassionate care to those who are affected by it. Our storied approach involves the sharing of narratives, both grand and personal, to engage students in pedagogical discourse promoting mastery of technical knowledge and ontological knowing. Our approach is presented in detail throughout the rest of the book, but at the heart of it is dialogue between students and text and other media and between people like faculty, clinicians, clients, friends, and family. We engage our students in conversation with those who have experienced the realities of perpetually living under the influence of illness.

We close this chapter with an introduction to Adrian and John, two visiting scholars who have graced our classroom with their presence since the beginning of our chronic illness courses. They play a key role in helping students put a face on chronic illness and thus more fully grasp the values that an Edgewood College education seeks to instill. Colleen has known them for over 20 years. Each has a diagnosis of HIV and, over the course of the illness, met the diagnostic criteria for AIDS. Adrian was diagnosed in 1984, John in 1992.

Three hundred sixty-three days a year John and Adrian live their conventional life—planting community gardens, tending to pets, and doing other community service, making accommodations as deemed necessary. However, twice annually they willingly come to class as representatives of "the disease of the day" to give a face to HIV and to inform our students' nursing practice. Their stories are shared in greater depth in chapter 4 and in the narratives provided in appendices F and G.

John and Adrian manage their chronic health issues (as John refers to them) from polar opposite perspectives. John is meticulous in his adherence to his medication regimen. Adrian takes "drug holidays" (or "structured treatment interruptions" as the medical community calls them) when side effects become too severe. Both responded differently in 1981 when news of a rare form of cancer was being reported among gay men. John writes, "My interpretation at hearing the news was that we *individually* were at risk. I think Adrian's response was more that our *community* was at risk."

Adrian began presenting his own lived experience to our class in 1994. John joined him in 1995. Their stories, as presented by them in class and written here, are testimony to the power of a storied approach, exemplifying the importance of whole-person care. John writes:

> When Adrian and I started speaking together regarding "Living with HIV" in a chronic health-issues class, I didn't realize I would end up talking about much more than AIDS. Who I am and how I respond to stress and crisis is a complex result of what I've experienced and learned over many years—my entire life. Which chronic condition is more important? Post traumatic stress disorder as a result of child sexual abuse? Attention deficit hyperactivity disorder? Chronic depression? AIDS? Can I separate them?
>
> I think it is important to realize when you are dealing with an individual with an illness, that they are so much more than their illness. Individuals carry their past and present on their shoulders.

One of the concepts discussed in our chronic illness courses is stigma. Although students can read the definition of stigma from a text and articulate an understanding of stigmatized individuals, Adrian best depicts his own lived experience with stigma in describing a visit to his dentist:

> I was flossing one night and pulled a cap off. I went to my longtime dentist to get it replaced, as he had done the original root canal and capping. I figured I had better tell him of my HIV status (that was the second big mistake of the week, the first was flossing). He pulled his hands out of my face and asked why I was there. It only made sense to me that I would come to him, but his thinking was, "Why would you throw money down a rat hole?" He was sure I would be dead before the glue dried.
>
> I didn't go back to a dentist until I found the AIDS Resource Center HIV Dental Clinic in Milwaukee. My fillings were falling out like mad. They knew it was a complication of my chemical cocktail, a potent combination of drugs I was taking. Wisely, they have hired a very personable, knowledgeable, and brutishly handsome dentist. Going to the dentist is something I look forward to even though he has done five root canals and caps.

Questions of truth, justice, compassion (or lack thereof), community, and partnership are all incorporated as John and Adrian explicitly portray living a life with chronic illness. Adrian describes losing his job, his health and life insurance, and his home, spending 3 years without any medical care and ultimately filing for bankruptcy. John shares his ongoing battle with post-traumatic stress disorder (PTSD) as a result of 8 years of childhood sexual abuse by his small town local dentist.

Collectively, they challenge our student's values and beliefs in discussing their lifelong experiences with discrimination as gay men. From John and Adrian, students learn about the complexity and tenuous nature of the phenomenon termed health, as well as about living a life.

Dr. Rachel Remen, noted author and medical educator, suggests, "Science is not a large enough metaphor to define life." Speaking to health care professionals, she submits, "life might be better defined by mystery" (Remen, 2003). In keeping with her wisdom, we employ our storied approach to teaching and learning about chronic illness management. We want our students to advance beyond factual knowledge to a rich, multifaceted appreciation of living a life with chronic illness and the mystery that surrounds it. In addition to learning more about John and Adrian in subsequent chapters, you will meet many others who have generously shared their stories with us—and now you—in order to promote quality care for those living a life with chronic illness.

REFERENCES

Ashe O. P., Sr. K. (2000, February). "Dominican Higher Education: Heritage and Challenge." Paper presented at Dominican College, Chicago IL. *At the heart of ministry is relationship: Sinsinawa Dominican Sponsorship.* (1999). Oak Creek WI.

Eby-Booth, R. (2003, Spring). The value of justice. *Edgewood College, The Magazine,* 60–63.

Edgewood College Undergraduate Catalogue (2002–2003). Madison WI.

Fields, J. (2003, Spring). The value of truth. *Edgewood College, The Magazine,* 4–9.

Heinen, N. (2003, Spring). The value of partnership. *Edgewood College, The Magazine,* 44–48.

Hopkins, O. P., Sr. M, & Naughton, O. P. Sr. S. (2003, Spring). The value of community. *Edgewood College, The Magazine,* 16–19.

Minden, P. (2003, Spring). Experiencing compassion. *Edgewood College, The Magazine,* 38–41.

Paynter O. P., Sr. M. (2002). *Phoenix from the fire: A history of Edgewood College.* Madison, WI: Edgewood College.

Reif, B. (2003, Spring). How do the young learn compassion? *Edgewood College, The Magazine,* 42–43.

Remen, R. N. (2003, September). *Keynote address.* Paper presented at HospiceCare's Eighth Annual End-of-Life Forum, Madison, WI.

3

Using Stories to Teach Whole-Person Care in Chronic Illness

As the principal faculty for teaching about chronic illness in Edgewood's nursing curriculum, we strive to instill in our students awareness of the many forms and outcomes of chronic illness, as well as to prepare them to intervene in its occurrence to minimize potential detriments. Colleen emphasizes its physical manifestations and Pamela its effects on the mind. These aspects inevitably overlap and intertwine with implications for social and spiritual health. We are vigilant in our efforts to neither demonize nor romanticize the experience of chronic illness and to find ways to convey Charmaz's message that chronic illness "means more than learning to live with it. It means struggling to maintain control over the defining images of self and over one's life. This struggle is grounded in concrete experiences of managing daily life, grappling with illness, and making sense of it" (1991, p. 5).

In order to help our students make sense of chronic illness and to further their development as thinkers and practitioners, we attempt to make as overt as possible the key assumptions underlying the content we teach. Nursing is holistic in its philosophical orientation, and the protection or restoration of health has been its primary goal. Edgewood's nursing curriculum (and thus the chronic illness courses) is rooted in this tradition, which holds that human beings are an integral part of nature, and that care in the face of disease and disability must consider the person in his or her entirety. A holistic perspective assumes that the whole has a unity, pattern, and uniqueness undiscoverable by examination of any one of its elements. The workings and characteristics of the whole are constantly emerging, and thus unpredictable. While the whole exerts power over its parts, the parts influence the whole. In a phrase, the whole is greater than the sum of its parts.

WHOLE-PERSON CARE

A holistic perspective is fundamental to the key supposition that chronic illness necessitates whole-person care. The phrase *whole-person care* can be ambiguous, mystifying, and fraught with New-Age stereotypes. In our curriculum, whole-person care is a kind of shorthand notation for the intersection of the six curricular strands: caring, health, client/person, professional nursing, environment, and critical thinking. In other words, it reminds us as educators that caring always occurs in a context and requires critical consideration of how numerous client, nurse, and environmental factors interact to promote and/or inhibit health. Whole-person care suggests an attitude, an overall approach to care, rather than any particular technique, and harkens back to Nightingale's vision of nursing.

Whole-person care presumes Minden's holistic depiction of health identified earlier in this chapter. That description accentuates the complex nature of health, which we sometimes try to simplify for our students by dissecting its physical, mental, social and spiritual facets. However, we acknowledge the paradox of doing so and reiterate that health is fragmented primarily in the minds of researchers and clinicians and for the convenience of learning. The word "health" itself derives from the same Indo-European root as heal, whole, and holy. "To be healthy is literally to be whole; to heal is to make whole" (Berry, 1995, p. 60). This understanding is foundational to our courses.

Whole-person care draws in part from principles of quantum thinking described by Wheatley (1999). An evolving worldview moving beyond the Newtonian logic that underlies all our modern institutions and accepts hierarchy, certainty, cause and effect relationships, either-or thinking, and a mechanistic view of the universe (Vella, 2002, p. 29) quantum thinking is informed by quantum physics. Quantum thinking considers the universe as composed of energy that is patterned and spontaneous and emphasizes the certainty of uncertainty, "both/and" thinking, and the interconnectedness of everything (Wheatley, 1999). In the quantum world, relationships are not just interesting, they are all there is to reality (Ibid. p. 34).

Earlier coursework in the sciences and nursing familiarizes students with the relationships between physiological systems within an individual. They enter the chronic illness courses with a sense of the mind-body connection, having learned that physical conditions can affect thinking, feelings, and even the spirit. Similarly, they recognize that when a person is hurting emotionally or spiritually, all sorts of physical ailments can crop up. Quantum thinking reinforces the integral nature of body, mind, milieu and spirit, and sets the stage for situating medical/ surgical and mental health content in the same chronic illness course. In our courses, students study the impact of chronic illness not only on the body and mind, but also on the social and spiritual integrity of afflicted individuals and of those caring for them. They explore the meaning of that experience from the client's perspective so that they might develop a capacity for forming therapeutic relationships that promote health even in the face of chronic illness.

A client is not just an abstract bio-psycho-social being, as many nursing texts suggest, but a real person "living a life" in a particular setting and set of circumstances. While care providers and academics (us included) often have elaborate theoretical definitions of health, we teach our students that from the perspective of those they will care for, "Health Is Success at Living" (Valliant, 1977, p. 366). In other words, persons with chronic illnesses tend to regard themselves as healthy to the extent that they are able to live as they desire.

Contemporary nursing has been defined primarily within the positivist tradition inherent in the biomedical model, but new science of the last several decades suggests that there is no neutral or objective perspective from which to capture what is real; thus, knowledge and truth are socially constructed rather than discovered. Nonetheless, nursing textbooks present facts that students often memorize, believing them to be absolutes. The facts appear as black-and-white options that conveniently omit reality. How students come to learn the application of these facts in the real world becomes the true test. "Nursing in the gray zone" is a phrase we use to describe the interface between what appear to be straightforward concrete facts with the realities of clients' lives. Quantum thinking suggests those realities are characteristically pluralistic and pliable.

Students do arrive in our courses with some predilection toward whole-person care, cultivated by their experiences in foundational liberal arts courses and the first two semesters of the nursing program. Though from the start they earnestly recite that health and illness can coexist and that nursing is both a science *and* an art, it takes the full semester for our students to grasp the profundity hidden in those words. Completing classes in the arts and humanities as well as the sciences has given them some awareness that knowledge evolves over time, but as a rule, when they ask nursing questions, they anticipate nominal, uncomplicated answers. At first, they have little tolerance for our frequent response: "It depends." Similarly, they often misconstrue our queries of them as seeking infallible replies. They assume that someone, usually us as the teachers, knows what is and is not real, and will reveal the universe's secrets if they just pay attention.

Although exasperating for students, "It depends" serves to reinforce the notion of whole person care by underscoring the importance of context in nursing practice. Nursing in the gray zone requires recognition that every client is unique and that the milieu in which he or she exists must be considered if any nursing intervention is to be effective. The milieu encompasses the physical and social resources and limitations that clients with chronic illnesses encounter and necessitates that students expand the notion of health care to include the sociopolitical realm of public policy. Considering context means recognizing that in spite of rampant medicalization, not all problems in life are health problems, and that there are vast varieties of therapeutic approaches within and beyond nursing that can help ameliorate concerns that are health related. At the most basic level, whole-person care is contingent on a humility that recognizes health, and what evokes or inhibits it, is sometimes a mystery.

Learning to provide whole-person care for people experiencing persistent health concerns obliges our students to reconstruct their understanding of health and health care. We ask them to see human health against a much more expansive and uncertain backdrop of global and ecological concerns. We encourage them to grapple with the intimate relationship between individual well being and community and environmental issues such as access to housing, transportation, food, and other resources. Expected to retain their grasp of clinical parameters like lab results, functional abilities, and physical assessment indicators, they must now consider them within the context of quality of life. They have to shift their emphasis from cure and quantity of life to focus on what it means to live a life.

Being faced with chronic illness requires coming to terms with one's limits, and as Charmez (1991) makes apparent, the sufferer can so readily become absorbed in the illness that she or he seems to become it. Care providers are at risk for sharing this misperception, especially when shame or disrepute accompanies the affliction, as is the case, for example, with AIDS or Schizophrenia. In the chronic illness courses we are continually challenged to find ways to engage our students in a process culminating not only in their possession of the necessary knowledge and skills for providing technically competent care but to transform their attitudes toward chronic illness and the people who live a life with it.

A STORIED APPROACH

Bruner (1986) delineates two distinctive ways in which we understand our world: the logico-scientific mode and the narrative mode. The first reflects positivism and seeks to establish universal truths through "tight analysis, logical proof, sound argument, and empirical discovery guided by reasoned hypothesis" (as cited in Schwandt, 1997, p. 99), while the later is concerned with the "storied nature of being" (Schwandt, 1997, p. 99). Both cognitive modes for ordering experience and constructing reality (Richardson, 1997, p. 28), each has different criteria for evaluating outcomes (Schwandt, ibid.). The ability to predict and control is key to the logico-scientific mode, whereas the narrative mode emphasizes the importance of understanding the meaning of certain social circumstances, events, roles, groups or interactions from the perspective of the participants involved (Denzin & Lincoln, 1994; Janesick, 1994; Locke, Spirduso, & Silverman, 1987). Drawing on the work of Donald Oliver, Vella uses different terms to characterize a similar split. She distinguishes between technical knowledge that is adaptive, publicly transferable information or skills, and ontological knowing that involves a diffuse apprehension of reality (Vella, 2002, p. 82).

Though the logico-scientific and narrative modes are irreducible to each other, they are complementary (Richardson, 1997, p. 28). This is the case as well with technical knowledge and ontological knowing. The purpose of the entire Edgewood nursing curriculum is to develop professional nurses who uphold the ideal of caring (Edgewood College Self Study Report, 1999, p. 9). Nursing action, that is, the treatment of human responses to actual and potential health threats, is the outcome of thinking. Our classes are premised on the notion that teaching and learning how to provide comprehensive care for the person experiencing chronic illness is facilitated by the integration of the logico-scientific and narrative modes and of technical knowledge and ontological knowing. In addition, we hold that knowing which mode is driving one's thought, the purpose for thinking and which mode best serves it, and what the consequences of one's cognitive processes are likely to be for themselves and those they serve is essential to providing whole-person care. Key to practicing nursing as an art is the ability to think in a variety of modes simultaneously.

The many technological advances enabled by the biomedical model cradled in the logico-scientific mode have certain value in whole person care, but these are always tempered by an appreciation for the innate healing capacity of human beings. In our classes, students are taught about the role of compassion and partnership in empowering clients to play a part in promoting their own health. With their modicum of objectivity the logico-scientific mode and technical knowledge bolster student courage and ability to *do for* clients what their chronic illnesses prohibit. The narrative mode and ontological knowing help them to simply *be with* clients when their subjective experience of living a life with chronic illness calls for that.

Because it was ingrained in them at least since primary school, our students are well versed in the logico-scientific mode. It has served them particularly well in earlier nursing coursework in which continual reinforcement of the importance of understanding human anatomy and physiology and knowing parameters for vital signs and lab values inadvertently fortifies the belief that being quantifiable is *the* mark of *reality*. To some extent, the chronic illness courses continue this trend, but now it is couched in an expectation that students develop a capacity for thinking in the narrative mode that rivals their facility with the logico-scientific mode.

A primary strategy we use to develop a narrative aptitude is to tell stories that blend objective and subjective knowing about chronic illness. These derive from our interactions with real people, including family, friends and acquaintances, colleagues, students, and those we serve. We share them only with explicit permission and without revealing identities except when authorized by those involved. We expose our students to relevant tales in scholarly texts and popular media and discuss their reactions. We have our students compose vignettes about circumstances in their own lives that are germane to chronic illness. Excerpts of each kind of these narratives appear later in this chapter and in subsequent chapters.

Another basic tactic is to pay close attention to the vocabulary used in the classroom and the clinical setting. Whether enfolded in a story, delivered in a typical academic lecture, or flowing freely in discussion, words have power that constructs reality. Words can promote under-standing and give a sense of order and control. They can facilitate health and therapeutic relationships by allowing us to describe phenomena or to identify and characterize problems. Likewise, they can have the opposite effect by focusing us only on problems or obscuring the measure of health that exists even in the worst pathology. Words used to classify diseases can be misconstrued to classify people (American Psychiatric Association, 1994), and inadvertently impose blame on affected individuals or conceal societal responsibility for human welfare. Labels used to designate populations incorrectly convey a sense of sameness. For example, "The use of the phrase 'the mentally ill' indirectly implies that all persons with a mental illness are alike and that the person's mental illness is all that needs to be known about him or her" (Taylor, 1993, p. 257).

While some words are relatively neutral or benign, we listen carefully for those that are affectively charged or part of what Ken Gergen terms the "language of deficit" (Cited in Hammond, 1998, p. 25). Exploring what words like *dysfunctional, co-dependent, stress, addiction, depressed,* and *burned out* (Hammond, 1998, p. 25) mean to our students helps to unveil their fears, biases, and misconceptions about working with people who have chronic illnesses.

The first days of the chronic illness courses begin a process of gently nudging students from their comfort with logico-scientific thinking and acute care into the gray zone of nursing, where the narrative mode is essential for grasping a given client's story. French philosopher Michel Foucault is often credited with saying, "Nothing is inherently evil, but everything is dangerous." So it goes with the logico-scientific mode. At times, especially when dealing with the physicality of the material world, it is efficacious to separate things into parts. Doing so facilitates understanding and can promote learning, especially for beginning nursing students. This becomes dangerous, however, when such a perspective is privileged over other ways of seeing.

The phrase, "Any way of seeing is also a way of not seeing," is a mantra of sorts introduced in earlier courses and chanted time and again in our theory and clinical course. We acknowledge here, and repeatedly to our students, that all vision is partial and situated. While the way we have shaped our curriculum allows certain leverage and flexibility in identifying what and how we will teach, it inevitably also creates blind spots that can be limiting. We persistently challenge our students to ask what is possible to know, to do, and to be given what they already are, do, know, and are being taught. We explore with them the social construction of the knowledge we teach, emphasizing that whatever seems natural, obvious, self-evident, or universal actually has a unique history and reason for being which can reveal much about society's power structure. What we come to take for granted or assume embodies particular values by determining what is or is not normal. Students come to our classes associating chronic illness with being abnormal and are often quite hesitant to care for individuals so branded.

We want students to be able to see their clients not as normal or abnormal, but as people, *whole* people. Because "What we see depends on our angle of repose" (Richardson, 1997, p. 92), we emphasize the importance of positioning the client at the forefront of care. We tell our students to "get the client's story" and explore the context in which it is rooted. Paradoxically, "The story of a life is less than the actual life, because the story told is selective, partial, contextually constructed and because the life is not yet over. But the story of a life is also more than the life, the contours and meanings allegorically extending to others, others seeing themselves, knowing themselves through another's life story, re-visioning their own, arriving where they started and knowing the place for the first time" (Richardson, 1997, p. 6).

LENSES TO LEARNING—ORGANIZING THEMES

In our classes, students learn that *both* scientific knowledge *and* empathic understanding of one's clients are essential to sound clinical judgement and skill. True empathy hinges on being able to fully understand the perspective of the person one seeks to help. We want our students not so much to do unto others as they would have others do unto them, as to do unto others as those others wish. This requires being able to perceive their clients clearly, which means gaining some aptitude for seeing the familiar as strange and the strange as familiar.

Students come to our classes fairly well versed in how to look for physical pathology, and this facilitates their learning about the impact of chronic illness on the body. They have less acuity, however, for distinguishing its more psychosocial-spiritual consequences and manifestations. To help magnify how all four facets of health are linked in the experience of chronic illness, we have mounted a trio of primary lenses in our teaching frame of whole-person care: self-regulation, stigma, and caregiver concerns.

A number of concepts could help elucidate the chronic illness experience. One of the most popular texts on the subject, Judith Miller's *Coping with Chronic Illness: Overcoming Powerlessness* (2002), addresses issues of empowerment, locus of control, and hopelessness. In the widely read *Chronic Illness: Impact and Interventions*, Lubkin and Larsen (2002) explore how a plethora of concerns such as chronic pain, altered mobility, fatigue, compliance, body image, advocacy, and social isolation figure in chronic illness. In our courses, we touch on each of these, but have found self-regulation, stigma, and caregiver concerns especially ideal organizing themes for the content presented in the chronic illness theory course, which is delineated in chapter 4. Patterned to some extent on the NCLEX blueprint, that content crosses over the boundaries of what was in an older curriculum thought of as two discrete courses in medical-surgical and psychiatric nursing. In our experience, the three lenses help expose commonalities and nuances in the various chronic conditions we explore no matter how the logio-scientifically oriented health care system diagnoses their associated symptoms, or whether their etiology is regarded as primarily physical or mental.

The Edgewood undergraduate nursing program prepares generalists for the field. Along with the curricular strands of caring, health, client/ person, professional nursing, environment, and critical thinking, the three lenses focus students on how chronic illness affects the lives their clients want to live. Similarly, the lenses bring to light how some aspects of the psychiatric and medical-surgical specialties are integral to all kinds of nursing. For example, all nurses, regardless of the setting in which they practice, need to be skilled in physical and mental status assessment.

Each of the lenses affords a novel slant on chronic illness, the person living a life with it, and whole-person care. In part, the self-regulation lens helps students deconstruct the biomedical model that spawns diagnostic tags and allows recognition of the important role of advocacy in nursing. Through the lens of stigma, students can begin to detect how stereotypical ideas about chronic illness negatively affect care. The caregiver concerns lens highlights both the strain chronic illness puts on personal and professional relationships, and the notion that caring for others is contingent on caring for oneself. Each new semester on the day the chronic illness theory course commences, we introduce incoming students to our trifocal teaching frame by telling several stories.

Ann's Story

Ann is a single woman approaching retirement. She lives alone in her own home and works as a professor in the city where she lives. Ann has many interests outside of work and spends little time at home. She owned a small black and white TV, limiting her reception to four or five local stations.

Ann's neighbors felt she was missing out by not having at least a VCR so that she could watch movies that might appeal to her. In addition, they regretted that she could not record selected programs while away at work or pursuing her other interests so she could enjoy them in her spare time. To remedy the obvious calamity Ann's clearly caring neighbors bought her a new color TV and VCR for Christmas. In addition, they purchased an entertainment center to house them.

Since Ann had a small home, there was limited space for the new furniture, necessitating considerable rearranging to accommodate the newly acquired gifts. A few weeks after Christmas, Ann commented to me that she was considering selling her piano to make room for all the new furniture. She regretted having to do this since her grandmother had brought it with her when she emigrated from Sweden many years before. However, with the large new TV and VCR, there simply was not enough room.

Ann felt awful about even mentioning what might be misconstrued an ungrateful complaint, especially considering how generous and thoughtful her neighbors had been. However, the gifts were more than she wanted, and now she was trying to figure out a way to give it back without insulting her neighbors or endangering their long friendship.

THE SELF-REGULATION LENS

Ann's story serves as a metaphor for what sometimes happens when a nurse cares for a client with a chronic illness. The client is living a life—*his or her* life—not the life the neighbors envision with a large TV and VCR. Sharing this story opens students to the possibility that they, as future nurses, might fall into the trap of presenting themselves as "the neighbors" when caring for individuals with chronic illness. The lens of self-regulation enlarges the picture of what it is like to be a client and reveals how clients and nurses can have parallel agendas. Nurses "know" what needs to be done and how to do it, and although well intended, they can often fall short of the mark, leaving clients metaphorically selling precious family heirlooms or, in reality, at odds with their health care providers, all in the name of good health care.

Conceptualization of self-regulation in the nursing literature ranges from a concrete mechanism characterized as the "Conscious control of various functions of the sympathetic nervous system" (Keegan, 1988, p. 197) to a complex theory explaining how illness beliefs centered on identity, time, cause, consequences, and cure or control influence health behavior (Berg, Evangelista, & Dunbar-Jacob, 2002, p. 208).

While the first formulation locates self-regulation within an individual, the later is predicated on a relationship, often between a client and a health care provider or system. In that scenario, self-regulation theory has been used to predict or promote *compliance. Compliance* is a catchall term, sometimes used synonymously with adherence, referring to how well a client maintains the therapeutic regimen set forth by his/her health-care providers. Its opposite, *noncompliance,* tends to have a harsh connotation, and the *noncompliant client* frequently is branded as unmotivated or manipulative.

In earlier courses, students learn about nursing in acute care settings. There, the lines of authority are fairly well defined, care provision is highly structured, and the hegemony of the biomedical model can manifest as paternalism. Though faculty have tried to instill the idea that trust is vital to therapeutic relationships, students arrive to study chronic illness having construed this to mean clients ought to follow their suggestions unconditionally. Nursing textbooks adamantly advise inclusion of the client in the plan of care, but hospitalization affords few options or opportunities for decision making that are not provider controlled. This biased and somewhat limited exposure to the concept of partnership is deceptive and misleading, leaving students ill prepared to deal with the complexities of chronic illness management. They assume that coveted techniques and skills learned and mastered in an acute care apply universally in all settings. Acclimated to the action-oriented role of the hospital-based nurse, students are prone to frustration, disappointment, and disillusionment when that restricted repertoire proves less necessary or valuable in caring for clients in long-term care facilities or at home.

Berg, Evangelista, and Dunbar-Jacob (2002) advise that "Compliance with medical recommendations is poor across all chronic disease regimens, which increases health care expenditures and prevents clients from achieving the full benefit of any intervention" (Berg, Evangelista, & Dunbar-Jacob, 2002, p. 203). While this may be true, Kirk (1990) and Primonmo (1989) note that research on the reasoning of chronic illness management from the viewpoint of those who have it suggests that professional care ought to be oriented to the needs of those with illness and not according to the expectations of professionals (cited in Thorne & Patersen, 1989, p. 175). Self-regulation theory recognizes clients as active participants in the process of managing health behaviors (Berg, Evangelista, & Dunbar-Jacob, 2002, p. 208).

The self-regulation lens keeps the focus on who it is that is living a life with chronic illness, thus putting the nurse in his/her place as a facilitator of client-desired change rather than as an enforcer of the care system's mandates for health. Self-regulatory models support maximum participation and decision-making on the part of the person living with chronic illness. Our students have to shift from a perception gained earlier of being "experts" who tell patients what to do to a perception of being informed practitioners who have something to offer only when they take the time to know their clients and collaborate with them (Minden, 2002). The gold standard is thus not adherence to a pre-scribed treatment devised by the medical profession but, rather, involvement in a partnership that allows the client to determine what is most in keeping with the kind of life s/he desires given the challenges of chronic illness.

Louie's Story

Louie has a very expressive face, with big, intense eyes that readily signal when he is feeling something deeply. When I ask him to describe himself, he says, "I guess the words that come to come to my mind are pretty liberal. I'd rather practice seeing the oneness in everything, rather than the differences." Louie will soon mark the beginning of his 12th year at Mendota. "I'll just say I am here for some serious reasons." Louie is certain he had a mental illness when he arrived at the Institute. "They termed it, initially, acute paranoid schizophrenia. . . . The most recent diagnosis is delusional disorder." He has taken psychotropic medications only for two brief periods. The first was about 8 years ago when "It was a situation of either take it or be put in a situation where I had to take it." A few months ago, of his own violation, he tried a new neuroleptic. It relaxed him, "as any sedative would, but I felt it was something I wanted to learn on my own and not have to depend on medication."

Whether Louie is currently mentally ill is contingent on how one perceives mental illness. "In terms of seeing everything in its proper perspective, no, I don't see everything in its proper perspective, most people don't." Nonethe-less, Louie is aware of a dramatic difference between the time he arrived at the Institute and now. "I'm healthier than I have ever been. I'm dealing with things now that I couldn't deal with in the past. . . . I have more control over my thinking. . . . I don't live with the fear and type of thoughts that I first had when I came here. . . . Am I mentally healthy? I can't exactly say. I have work to do, but I can say I am nothing like I was in the past." It is likely that Louie will never be allowed to leave Mendota. "There is a possibility that I may never leave. . . . I don't know. I'm not overly worried about it. My main concern is just finding peace and contentment within myself. That process is happening, and that is the most important thing."

The belief that there is *something greater* than himself is key to Louie's conception of health. "I think to be healthy basically means to be light. To be able to incorporate all the emotions. To be able to feel everything and not be necessarily controlled by everything. . . . To be healthy means to be in love, not so much with something on the outside, as with inside . . . loving yourself. Not your body or your mind or your thoughts. Loving that in you which is love." Louie often uses the inflection of his deep voice, or thoughtful pauses to emphasize his feelings. "Being healthy is being fearless. . . . If you feel fear you don't let it control you. Being healthy is living the best type of life you can lead. Eating foods that are good for you. Exercising. Thinking good thoughts. Not letting the bad thoughts come in and take over. . . . So it just comes down to being light, and when you feel serious, to be light anyway. There is nothing wrong with being serious, but to be dragged down by it, depressed, or just terribly unhappy, that's not healthy. Seeing the positive in everything, looking at everything as an opportunity, that's being healthy."

Health goes beyond the individual to people in interaction. "Like Bradshaw says, dysfunction comes out in relationships, not when you all are out hanging out by yourself." Healthy interaction is characterized by "thoughtfulness, gentleness, respect." Health derives from the "something greater" that Louie alluded to earlier. "I think the bottom line is what we call God, some people say the Higher Power. That's the ultimate . . . Have that and everything else takes care of itself. . . . People come and people go, but the love of the Higher Power doesn't budge. It's always faithful. And getting to know that is more important than anything for me. . . . Everything happens the way it is supposed to happen. This earthly life is temporal. I am more than this body. I am not my mind, thoughts, or emotions. There is just something greater than that, within me." (Excerpted from Minden, 1999, pp. 394–401.)

THE STIGMA LENS

Mendota is a state mental health facility with a large inpatient forensic psychiatric population. It is a rare student who knows it as anything other than a shadowy place where the patients are not only "crazy" but also have committed significant crimes. Our students' discomfort is palpable as we begin to tell Louie's story, perhaps because they fear they will encounter him, or someone like him in the chronic illness clinical course. It is quickly apparent that they have difficulty reconciling their preconceived negative images of psychiatric patients with Louie's eloquent description of health, and at the conclusion, their questions betray that they think he is both highly intelligent and must have been mistakenly detained. Their reactions let slip a proclivity towards believing that one or several bad deeds defines the person and that chronic illness annihilates the possibility of concurrent health. They reveal as well a tendency to equate chronic illness with hopelessness and skepticism toward the human capacity for change. Their way of seeing blinds them. "Normality is never recognized by the attendant in a milieu where abnormality is the normal expectancy" (Goffman, 1961, p. 85).

Care-provider attitude is a determinant of client response to treatment and rehabilitation (Keane, 1991), and a caring attitude seems to lead to greater improvement than does indifference (Forchuk et al., 1998). Client unpopularity, as perceived by the nurse, has negative consequences for both the care provider and the recipient (Kus, 1994). Attributions of low social value or moral worth, undesired stigma, "own fault" diagnoses, fear-causing conditions, negative patient behavior, and incompetence on the part of the nurse are all causes of patient unpopularity (Kus, 1994). The clinical experiences offered in NRS 341 are ripe with all these potentialities for students to dislike the clients.

All too often, students arrive in a new course encumbered by a load of baggage that impedes their willingness to experiment with new ideas and behaviors. In the case of the courses we teach, a common impediment is a mentality of US (the young, well, strong, and resourceful caregivers), and THEM (the old, sick, weak, and poor care recipients). This is complicated further by the fact that in the clinical course, THEM includes clients who are physically handicapped or deformed due to injury, illness, or aging, and/or are perceived to have character flaws assumed inherent in conditions like AIDS, liver disease, or mental illness. The socioeconomic backgrounds of a number of the clients varies quite substantially from those of many students, and it is not uncommon for students to hold unconscious prejudice against clients of a different class, race, religion, or nationality. Diagnoses of personality or substance abuse disorders are fairly prevalent among the clients, and students easily construe these to be the result of behaviors under their control. It is easy as well for them to judge those clients who have criminal histories as socially and morally inferior.

We share Louie's story in the theory course because not only does it beautifully express our understanding of health, but it also conveys the reality that a number of clients that students will care for in the clinical course bear highly stigmatized conditions and characteristics. The word "stigma" derives from the Greek verb *stizein*, which means to tattoo. Chronic illness, especially chronic mental illness, can leave a mark of disgrace or reproach. Once labeled with a mental illness, "everything you do gets understood in reference to your illness" (Deegan,

1993, p. 9). In Louie's words, "You have this label, stigma on you. Crazy person. I mean the shame . . . I'm labeled for the rest of my life, I'm no good" (Minden, 1999, p. 399).

A small percentage of students new in the chronic illness courses have prior experience in long-term care, but far fewer have ever even been in a psychiatric setting. Stigmatized individuals or populations can create caregiver anxiety by threatening one's values and sense of security. Encounters with physically or mentally challenged individuals call attention to the fact that life is not always fair, and this brings students face-to-face with their own vulnerability and mortality. Classroom instruction in how to deal with potentially manipulative and violent behavior, coupled with occasional inappropriate or negative client conduct, reinforces their mistaken sense that the most important psychiatric nursing skill is self-defense.

When they enter our classes a lot of students express disinterest in dealing with the old or the dying, and most express total terror at the prospect of caring for *"schizophrenics, manic-depressives, or drug abusers."* They do not yet know that in their presence most clients will manifest remarkably pleasant and positive demeanors. Once accustomed to looking through the lens of stigma, most students will become caregivers who value and respect chronically ill clients as remarkable people who are doing the best they can to face with dignity their aging, a disease process, or the end of life.

Roy's Story

The old man could not speak. Strokes had affected both sides of his body, so that he could move his arms and hands only with difficulty and within a limited range. His body and limbs had become permanently curled from disuse, and could not be straightened. He was lifted to a chair, and back to bed, as the care plan dictated. When I met him, he was fed pureed food from a spoon that an aide or orderly inserted in his mouth. His lower body was wrapped in a large towellike blanket, which could be easily changed when he wet himself.

He taught me that he could feed himself if I bent the spoon a certain way and placed it in his good hand, and that this was important to him. He taught me that he could use a urinal, and that I could recognize his need before he wet himself. He taught me that he looked and felt better in trousers. At the end of one shift, he held my hand, and looked at me. His grip was strong and his gaze was clear. His hands and eyes said to me that we had worked together well.

He spoke to me in words only once, when I gave him grapefruit juice. "Goddamn, son of a bitch," he said. I learned that he did not like grapefruit juice. I learned also that some words are stored apart from and more deeply than the others and are kept for special need.

After a time, the old man got pneumonia. The doctor (on the telephone—doctors did not like to come to that place) and the nurses and the care plan said that he must be bathed in cold water and alcohol to reduce his fever. They said that he must be turned on his stomach, his head over the side of the bed, and his back must be pounded to dislodge mucous from his lungs. They said that his temperature must be taken, and that if he did not hold the thermometer in his mouth, it must be inserted in his rectum. They said that if he did not drink, fluids must be given to him through needles and tubes. His eyes said no, but the nurses said it must be done. I obeyed the nurses. His hands fought, and I tied them with cloth restraints to the metal rails of his bed. After that, his eyes looked through me to the cream-colored walls, and said nothing.

The old man died on someone else's shift. It did not occur to me to come and be with him. It would have seemed strange to the nurses and other workers if I had been in that place when I was not being paid. I saved, and still have, a small, rectangular block of rubber that the old man left behind. It is rounded on one long side to fit the palm and thumb and has four dents on the other long side to fit the fingers. It is used to strengthen the grip of a man's hand. (Froemming, 1990)

THE CAREGIVER CONCERNS LENS

Dealing effectively with chronic illness requires a comprehensive continuum of care that often positions the ill person's significant others as caregivers. The expression caregiver refers to anyone, paid or not, who assists someone else who is to some degree incapacitated and needs help (Family Caregiver Alliance, 2001). Estimates of the number of caregivers in the United States vary greatly depending on how the term is defined and the criteria used (Ibid). Just a sampling of statistics extrapolated from many cited in the Family Caregiver Alliance's *Fact Sheet: Selected Caregiver Statistics* (2001) help illuminate the extent of family caregiving and the challenges it creates:

1) Fifty-two million informal and family caregivers provide care to someone aged 20+ who is ill or disabled. Among those caring for family or friends aged 65+, two thirds report having to rearrange work schedules, decrease work hours, or take an unpaid leave to meet these responsibilities. Thirty-one percent of those

caring for persons aged 65+ describe their own physical health as "fair to poor" (Health and Human Services, June 1998).

2) Nearly one in every four households (22.4 million) is involved in caregiving to persons aged 50+, and this number is estimated to reach 39 million by 2007. Just over half of the involved caregivers are employed full-time and almost two-thirds are employed either full- or part-time. Caregivers of people aged 50+ spend an average of 17.9 hours per week providing care, and 20 hours per week for individuals aged 65+. Caregivers spend an average of 4.5 years proving care (National Alliance for Caregiving and AARP, 1997).

3) Approximately 75% of those providing care to older family members and friends are female (Health and Human Services, 1998; National Alliance for Caregiving and AARP, 1997) and even though some studies show a relatively equitable distribution of caregiving between men and women, female caregivers spend 50% more time providing care than male caregivers (Health and Human Services, 1998).

4) A study of elderly spousal caregivers (aged 66–96) (cited in Family Caregiver Alliance, 2000) found that caregivers who experience mental or emotional strain have a 63% higher risk of dying than do noncaregivers, and caregivers use prescription drugs for depression, anxiety, and insomnia two to three times as often as the rest of the population.

Decreased family size, increased numbers of women in the workforce, and increased longevity all tax the ability of the American family to continue a long history of caring for its members, young and old in health or sickness, mostly independently. Whole-person care in the event of incurable long-term health problems compels students to look beyond individual clients to the physical and social milieu in which they exist. Just at the point where they finally feel a sense of comfort *doing for* patients in acute care settings, we ask our students to learn how to *be with* clients, often on their own turf, and to expand their understanding of client to include a family or a group.

In our classes, students learn about role changes not only for the chronically ill person, but also for all those trying to care for him or her. They will come to know first hand and in a very experiential manner about the burden, isolation, uncertainty and fear, physical and emotional stress, and the burnout that often accompanies caregiving.

The caregiver lens helps them to see the importance of client education, advocacy, and developing active partnerships with those they hope to help. Carrying out these responsibilities requires a firm hold on therapeutic boundaries.

Roy's story underscores how thoughtfully and tenderly one needs to traverse the boundaries of care. It highlights, as well, what we know from personal experience and the nursing literature. Stress is inherent in our chosen profession (Gallagher, 1989; Hinshaw & Atwood, 1983; Huber, 1994; Kramer & Schmalenberg, 1991; Lyon & Werner, 1987; McCranie, Lambert, & Lambert, 1987). The current nursing shortage, rotating shifts, physical demands of providing direct care, difficulties in communication, and a plethora of other challenges impinge on the nurse's ability to care for clients, let alone himself or herself. Pain and suffering as well as death and dying are common sequelae of chronic illness. Constant exposure to trauma and tragedy in the lives of others is a formidable threat to a nurse's well being. Witnessing, at times powerlessly, catastrophic events in the lives of others shatters the illusion of one's own invulnerability (Davidson & Jackson, 1985).

As hard as it is for our students to continually shift their view from client to caregiver and from concrete needs to more amorphous ones, it is even more onerous for them to focus their sight on themselves as professional caregivers. The caregiver lens magnifies the paradoxical nature of practice for the nurse in the arena of chronic illness. Whole-person care mandates that the caregiver maintain a global perspective over a vast scope of external concerns, while also engaging in intense introspection and attention to personal need. It requires being fully present to clients without wearing martyrdom like a merit badge. In short, whole-person care is contingent on caring for self and requires a stance of detached concern. A solid knowledge base and sharp skills are essential, but they have value only in the context of knowing one's place as a caregiver. As Maradee, one of our students turned coteacher who the reader will learn more about in chapters 4 and 5, put it, "it is important to recognize that you are only a second in the client's life, but an important second."

CONCLUSION

By the time they leave the chronic illness courses, we expect our students to be familiar with and comprehend contemporary research and information relevant to chronic illness and to know that empirical generalizations can never express the depth and breadth of what it means to live a life with chronic illness. They need to recognize that people always precede and exceed any diagnostic labels applied to them, and that each person's illness experience is unique. The chronic illness courses are all about deepening students' understanding of caring, health, client/person, professional nursing, environment, and critical thinking in order to create a sufficient ability to practice nursing in the gray zone and tolerate the ambiguity of an answer like *it depends*. We have no aspirations of turning every student into a nurse as passionate about caring for individuals with chronic illness as we are. We do, however, want to help them see beyond their initial stereotypical view of the hopelessness of chronicity and long-term care.

In our classes, students, teachers, and clients share their stories toward the end of enhancing nursing care in the event of chronic illness. The following chapters elaborate how we go about doing that.

REFERENCES

American Psychiatric Association. (1994). *Diagnostic and statistical manual of mental disorders* (4rd ed.). Washington, DC: American Psychiatric Association.

Berg, J., Evangelista, L. S., & Dunbar-Jacob, J. M. (2002). Compliance. In I. M. Lubkin & P. D. Larsen (Eds.), *Chronic illness: Impact and interventions* (pp. 203–232). Boston: Jones and Bartlett Publishers.

Berry, W. (1995). Health is membership. *UTNE Reader*, Sept./Oct., 60–63.

Bruner, J. (1986). *Actual minds, possible worlds*. Cambridge, MA: Harvard University Press.

Byrne, R. (1984). *The other 637 best things anybody ever said*. New York: Fawcett Crest.

Charmez, K. (1991). *Good days, bad days*. New Brunswick, NJ: Rutgers University Press.

Davidson, P., & Jackson, C. (1985). *The nurse as a survivor: Delayed post-traumatic stress reaction and cumulative trauma in nursing* (pp. 1–13). Pergamon Press.

Deegan, P. (1993). Recovering our sense of value after being labeled. *Journal of Psychosocial Nursing, (31)*4, 7–11.

Denzin, N. K., & Lincoln, Y. S. (1994). Introduction, entering the field of qualitative research. In N. K. Denzin & Y. S. Lincoln (Eds.), *Handbook of qualitative research* (pp. 1–17). Thousand Oaks, CA: Sage Publications.

Edgewood College Department of Nursing. (1999). *Self study report*. Madison, WI: Edgewood College.

Family Caregiver Alliance. (October, 2001). Fact Sheet: Selected Caregiver Statistics. *http://www.caregiver.org/factsheets/selected_caregiver_statistics.html*. Retrieved 6/17/03.

Froemming, R. (1990). Untitled. Unpublished manuscript.

Forchuk, C., Westwell, J., Martin, M. L., Azzapardi, W. B., Kosterewa-Tolman, D., & Hux, M. (1998). Factors influencing movement of chronic psychiatric patients from the orientation to the working phase of the nurse-client relationship on an inpatient unit. *Perspectives in Psychiatric Care, 34*(1), 36–44.

Gallagher, D. (1989). Is stress ripping nurses apart? *Imprint, 36*(2), 59–63.

Goffman, E. (1961). *Asylums. Essays on the social situation of mental patients and other inmates.* Garden City, NY: Doubleday.

Hammond, S. A. (1998). *Appreciative inquiry.* Plano, TX: Thin Book Publishing Co.

Hinshaw, A. S., & Atwood, J. R. (1983). Nursing staff turnover, stress, and satisfaction: Models, measures, and management. In H. H. Werley & J. J. Fitzpatrick (Eds.), *Annual review of nursing research* (pp. 133–153). New York: Springer Publications.

Huber, D. G. (1994). What are the sources of stress for nurses? In J. McCloskey & H. K. Grace (Eds.), *Current issues in nursing* (pp. 623–631). St. Louis: Mosby.

Janesick, V. J. (1994). The dance of qualitative research design. Metaphor, methodolatry and meaning. In N. K. Denzin & Y. S. Lincoln (Eds.), *Handbook of qualitative research* (pp. 209–219). Thousand Oaks, CA: Sage Publications.

Keane, M. (1991). Acceptance vs. Rejection: Nursing students' attitudes about mental illness. *Perspectives in Psychiatric Care, 27*(3), 13–18. (Chap. 1).

Keegan, L. (1988). Relaxation: Opening the door to change. In B. M. Dossey, L. Keegan, C. E. Guzzetta, & L. G. Kolkmeier (Eds.), *Holistic nursing* (pp. 195–222). Gaithersburg, MD: Aspen Publications.

Kirk, K. (1990). *Chronically ill patients' perceptions of nursing.* Unpublished master's thesis. University of Saskatchewan, Saskatoon, SK. Canada.

Kramer, M., & Schmalenberg, C. (1991). Job satisfaction and retention, insights for the 90's, Part 1. *Nursing 91, 21*(3), 50–55.

Kus, R. J. (1994). Nurses and unpopular clients. In J. McCloskey & H. K. Grace (Eds.), *Current issues in nursing* (pp. 671–675). St. Louis: Mosby.

Leonard, J. (2002). The value of compassion. *Edgewood College—The Magazine.* Winter, 4–7.

Locke, L. F., Spirduso, W. W., & Silverman, S. J. (1987). *Proposals that work. A guide for planning dissertations and grant proposals* (2nd ed.). Newbury Park: Sage Publications.

Lubkin, I. M., & Larsen, P. D. (Eds.). (2002, 5th ed.). *Chronic illness: Impact and interventions.* Boston: Jones and Bartlett Publishers.

Lyon, B. L., & Werner, J. S. (1987). Stress. In J. J. Fitzpartick & R. L. Taunton (Eds.), *Annual review of nursing research* (pp. 3–32). New York: Springer Publications.

McCranie, E., Lambert, V., & Lambert, C. (1987). Work stress, hardiness and burnout among hospital staff nurses. *Nursing Research, 36*(6), 374–377.

Miller, J. (2000). *Coping with chronic illness: Overcoming powerlessness.* Philadelphia: F. A. Davis.

Minden, P. (1999). *Nursing a sense of humor.* Unpublished doctoral dissertation. University of Wisconsin, Madison.

Primomo, J. (1989). *Patterns of chronic illness management, psychosocial development, family and social environment and adaptation among diabetic women.* Unpublished doctoral dissertation. University of Washington, Seattle, Washington.

Richardson, L. (1997). *Fields of play. Constructing an academic life.* New Brunswick, NJ: Rutgers University Press.

Schwandt, T. A. (1994). Constructivist, interpretivist approaches to human inquiry. In N. K. Denzin & Y. S. Lincoln (Eds.), *Handbook of qualitative research* (pp. 118–137). Thousand Oaks, CA: Sage Publications.

Schwandt, T. A. (1997). *Quality inquiry.* Thousand Oak, CA: Sage Publications.

Thorne, S., & Paterson, B. (1998). Shifting images of chronic illness. *Image: Journal of Nursing Scholarship, 30*(2), 173–178.

Valliant, G. E. (1977). *Adaptation to life.* Boston: Little, Brown and Company.

Vella, J. (2002). *Learning to Listen, Learning to Teach: The Power of Dialogue in Educating Adults.* San Francisco: Jossey-Bass.

Wheatley, M. J. (1999). *Leadership and the new science.* San Francisco: Berrett-Koehler.

Teaching the Theory Component

Understanding the conceptual considerations of chronic illness assists in developing an appreciation for the unique role nurses assume in providing care to persons living a life with chronic illness. This chapter discusses classroom implementation and thus focuses on teaching the theory and academic content of chronic illness.

LETTING GO OF CONTENT

Our theory course (NRS 340) is a four-credit course with classes that meet for 2 hours twice a week over 16 weeks. The course is designed to meet five objectives that derive from and are intertwined with the six curricular strands: caring, health, client/person, professional nursing, environment, and critical thinking.

Course Objectives

1. Examine the concept of chronicity and characteristics of specific chronic illnesses.
2. Examine the interplay between the client with a chronic illness and the environment in which they exist.
3. Identify resources that have been developed to aid individuals and families who have chronic illnesses.
4. Discuss management of chronic health problems within the framework of caring.
5. Integrate nursing science with an understanding of the lived experience of individuals and families living with chronic illness

The course objectives serve as a compass, continually directing us to the place the course has in the overall curriculum, so as not to overlap with the content addressed in earlier or subsequent courses. In other words, the objectives guide what gets *covered* in the course.

Somewhere around the time we were revising the undergraduate program, the Edgewood nursing faculty attended a weekend conference presented by world-renowned educator Richard Paul. Excited and rejuvenated by his work, we left vowing to completely overhaul our theory courses and revitalize classroom teaching. Though our always too-busy academic schedules intervened in ways that precluded total transformation, we did learn a very important lesson from Dr. Paul that has had a profound effect on how we think about our curriculum and teaching. When we are feeling particularly overwhelmed by the ever increasing amount of material our profession and accreditation agencies expect us to disseminate to students, we comfort ourselves with Dr. Paul's wise challenge to "let go of content." This was such a refreshing idea, though initially quite frightening.

Clearly, a history professor can eliminate a battle here or a treaty there or a literature professor might omit a novel or short story, but how could nursing instructors possibly omit anything? We felt compelled to cover everything! After all, our students would be taking care of real patients, sometimes in life or death situations. Paul's "let go" sparked many heated debates among faculty about what it means to cover a topic. We heard faculty say they threw out certain exam questions because they "didn't cover it in class." Was a topic covered because the instructor mentioned it in class? There is something incongruous with this line of reasoning, and it prevented us from letting go of content. It is easy to translate the ever expanding body of nursing knowledge to mean, "we have more material to 'cover' in class." Paul's legacy for our course has been our commitment to continually question and revise as needed what we teach and how we do it. Several other caveats that have given us permission beyond Paul's to let go of content follow.

LIMITED LANGUAGE AND PARADOXICAL PEDAGOGY

As teachers our job is not merely to feed our students digestible bites of knowledge and evaluate their ability to regurgitate them but, rather, to engage them in a process of discovery that clarifies, edifies, and creates meaning that ultimately enhances their practice. This is contingent not only on *their* readiness to learn but also on our own. One thing we learn over and over again is that there are limits to language.

Our philosophy of *whole person care* and a *storied approach* to teaching are intended to foster in our students an ability to think in a variety of modes simultaneously. Trying to sum our selves and actions as teachers in a book or a chapter, much less in singular phrases, is indeed challenging. Once represented by particular names, phenomena become inextricably snarled in the nuances that accompany them. Various meanings of the words used, images peculiar to them at any particular time, theories that have incorporated them, and their emotional or political context can spin out further webs of terminology that can catch us in a terminal snare (Miller & Dzurec, 1993). The language we use both allows us to and prevents us from adequately expressing what it is we teach and how we do it. Sometimes words confound us with their multiple meanings.

Pamela's Humbling Experience

About my fourth year into teaching, I found myself especially overextended in my work commitments. A propensity toward perfectionism was beginning to do me in. The hours I was spending trying to come up with a faultless lesson in every class every week was leading me down the path toward what is often called burnout. One of my students, a "mature learner" in her 30s who had returned for a second degree, astutely noted, "You look awful. I think you need some time off." I confessed to being stressed and that my husband was getting sick of taking a second place to The Academy.

As her advisor and teacher for three of the courses she had taken, I had come to know Heather fairly well. To support herself through her studies, she worked as a nanny, and she was also a substitute teacher in the preschool where my daughter was enrolled. Thus, she knew not only me, but also my family. In what was clearly her fondness for us, she insisted that I allow her to baby sit so my husband and I could have an evening of respite. After agonizing over whether that would constitute a transgression of the student-teacher relationship, I finally relented by insisting that I would take her up on her offer as long as she would allow me to pay her.

My husband and I indulged in a rather extravagant evening and had a lovely time. When we returned home I told Heather about the expensive restaurant where we had dined. I teasingly tried to play on her sympathies. "I'm feeling much more relaxed, but I hope you won't add to my stress by charging us too much. You know I'm just a poor teacher."

"Yes," Heather replied. "I know, I've had you for three classes!"

Another recurrent lesson for us is that humility is an essential ingredient for survival in academia. We take our teaching seriously, but we take ourselves lightly. We do not and cannot know everything our students need to know. Ellsworth (1997, p. 9) notes the essentially paradoxical nature of pedagogy and challenges us to consider what we might learn from ways of teaching that are predicated on the ironic impossibility of teaching. No matter how well intentioned or planned, our curriculum always misses its mark to some degree. We each have own teaching styles, as do the guest lecturers who grace our classroom, but the transcendence of our pedagogical framework—that is, the whole-person care frame and its three lenses—gives some constancy and cohesion to what otherwise might be a chaotic classroom.

On a regular basis, we also have to relearn that all understanding is incomplete and/or fleeting. We recognize that reduction of thinking into two camps is simplistic. Within the logico-scientific and the narrative modes, or the technical knowledge and ontological knowing dichotomy, one could find the four fundamental patterns of knowing in nursing conceptualized by Carter years ago (cited in Chinn & Kramer, 1999). Empirical knowing with its devotion to sensory experience springs from the logico-scientific mode and is consistent with technical knowledge. Aesthetic, ethical, and personal knowing flow more readily with the narrative mode and ontological knowing. At the most basic level, we are trying to teach our students to think like a nurse. This means appreciating that some things are inexplicable or unknowable (Silva, Sorrell, & Sorrell, 1995), and that unknowing can be a pattern of knowing (Munhall, 1993). Knowing what to call our teaching principles is simply a guide to using them intentionally (Vella, 2002, p. 227).

A WEB OF WHAT AND HOW

As the primary faculty we are to a large extent accountable for what happens in the theory course. Like Vella, we understand accountability to be a mutual process that means, "the teacher is responsible to teach what he has promised learners will learn" and "the learners are responsible to do the work of learning" (2002, p. 213). In our case the teachers' promise is encapsulated in the course objectives, and at every turn, we must consider how to determine whether our students are fulfilling their end of the academic bargain.

Student Assessment

In order to pass the theory course, each student must demonstrate mastery of the scientific knowledge necessary to provide competent care to individuals with chronic illness. It is undeniable that nursing practice relies to a large extent on hard data. The purpose of the NCLEX-RN (National Council Licensure Exam) is to determine whether a given applicant is minimally safe to practice nursing. We appraise this primarily through four NCLEX-like multiple-choice exams. In order to familiarize the students with our testing format, the first exam is a take home. The next two exams are completed in class, with the third including questions about material introduced subsequent to the second exam and topics addressed in all previous classes. In other words, the third exam is comprehensive. Three fourths of a student's final grade derives from his or her score on these three exams. The standardized, commercially prepared, and Web-based fourth exam is not graded, but it is required for completion of the course. It helps students to gauge their strengths and weaknesses related to the NCLEX and provides aggregated data for the purpose of program evaluation.

Though we are adamant that we will not "teach to the NCLEX," and our test questions theoretically require not only memorization of facts but clinical judgment, we admit that they in no way assess the depth or breadth of our students' ontological knowing. Fortunately, the close contact we have with them during clinical experiences, as discussed in chapter 5, allows us greater opportunity for that. We take great pains to let our students know the limits of our assessment methods and how such tests can inadvertently undermine they ability to practice nursing in the grey zone. While an answer of "it depends" followed by sound options and rational is often applauded in the clinical arena, it is never a plausible response on the NCLEX or our exams. We tell our students up front that there will always be one right answer for every NCLEX or class exam question. We discuss strategies for discerning the best response, even when they know that in the real world "it depends" is the superior answer.

To preclude student grades from hinging solely on test performance, we also give credit toward the final grade for work done in advance of each class. Colleen uses the student study guide that accompanies the medical-surgical nursing text toward this end, along with a selection of clinical simulations available on CD-ROM. Pamela has created a series of worksheets corresponding in part to the psychiatric nursing text and other materials, which are discussed later in this chapter. Students are awarded a set number of points for each assignment handed in prior to the class period in which the relevant topic is being addressed. Partial points may be granted in the event that the work is incomplete or inaccurate. We have found this method particular useful in motivating our students to complete assigned readings in a timely fashion. Though optional, the weekly assignments give students an opportunity to earn the equivalence of on exam's worth of points toward their final grade.

What we actually teach—the content—and how we go about doing it—the process—constantly evolves. Below, we identify some of the basics of each, recognizing that, though we address them separately here, in the classroom they are intimately intertwined.

Content—The *What* of Our Teaching

As noted earlier, the theory course situates what customarily might be regarded as medical/surgical and psychiatric/mental health content in one chronic illness course founded on the notion of whole-person care. Because we are still "old school" enough to worry about our students' passing their board exams, that content derives to a substantial degree from the topics outlined in the NCLEX blueprint. Table 4.1 delineates what we teach in the class. That listing of topics might falsely simplify what are really very complex issues, but it helps us organize the semester. In general, there is one class period dedicated to each topic listed. In the course syllabus and schedule, each topic is prefaced with "Nursing Care of the Client With . . . " We do this to remind the students that they are learning to care for people, not medical conditions.

At first glance, the topics presented in Table 4.1 probably make this class look like other, more conventional nursing courses. Even were the reader to scrutinize the syllabus our students receive each semester, what is unique about the course might not be readily apparent. While we maintain that teaching nursing care of people living with chronic illness is very different than teaching acute care, we use the very same medical-surgical nursing, psychiatric nursing, pharmacology, and nutrition textbooks that are required for students in their previous adult health classes (NRS 310/311). The decision to do so was not made simply to prevent further student disinterest in chronic illness management by having them spend another $100–$200 on additional textbooks.

Each year, the nursing faculty as a whole decides collaboratively on which primary texts to use in each course. Though these change from year to year to keep up with continual shifts in information and practice, they are selected from the usual menu of conventional reference books that nursing faculty are inundated with annually. We have found them

TABLE 4.1 NRS 340 Content

Medical-Surgical Nursing	Psychiatric Nursing
Nursing Care of the Client With Chronic Illness Introduction to the Self-regulation, Stigma, and Caregiver Lenses	
Metabolic problems and self-regulation Case model: Diabetes mellitus and self	Chronic mental illness Case model: Social construction of stigma
Sensory/perceptual disorders Case model: CVA/Parkinson's	Psychotic disorders Case model: Schizophrenia
Changes in mobility and self-image Case models: MS, ALS, and MG	Mood disorders Case models: Depression & mania
Brain insult Case models: Dementia & TBI	Safety concerns Case model: Restraints and seclusion
GI disorders Case model: Crohn's disease	Iatrogenic disease Case model: Psychopharmacology
Changes in cardiac function Case models: CHF and hypertension	Substance-related disorders Case model: Multiple substance abuse
Changes in oxygenation Case model: COPD	Anxiety disorders Case model: ODC
Changes in mobility and self-image Case models: Arthritis and osteoporosis	Personality disorders Case models: Obsessive-compulsive, narcissistic, borderline, antisocial personalities
Changes in immunocompetence Case model: AIDS	Dissociative disorders Case models: PTSD and DID
Changes in energy levels & quality of life Case model: Chronic renal failure	Eating disorders Case models: Anorexia, bulimia, obesity
Changes in energy levels & quality of life Case model: Chronic liver failure	Mental disorders of childhood or adolescence Case models: ADHD and autism
Facing the end of life Case model: Family caregiver concerns	Facing the end of life Case model: Professional caregiver concerns

quite adequate in terms of addressing the logico-scientific, technical knowledge our students need to care for clients with chronic illness. Each topic area delineated in Table 4.1 has corresponding readings in these texts that help ready students for classroom discussion.

Where the course syllabus hints at what is unique about NRS 340 is that the concept of tertiary prevention directs the selection and presentation of content. Tertiary prevention emphasizes nursing management outside the acute care setting and provides students with valuable information regarding the nurse's role. The venue of preparatory materials listed in the syllabus comes not only from the required texts but is balanced with selections from Charmez's *Good Days, Bad Days*, articles culled from the current literature, the books *Tuesdays With Morrie* and *Gracefully Insane*, and both educational and popular videos. These all help put students in the narrative frame of mind necessary for ontological reflection on what it means to live a life with chronic illness.

Process—The How of Our Teaching

A primary challenge for any faculty member teaching chronic illness management and whole-person care lies in shifting the content emphasis from acute care interventions to living a life. For example, when we discuss nursing care of clients with changes in cardiac function, very little time is spent discussing inpatient management for an acute episode of heart failure, which is likely to be 2 or 3 days in length. Rather, the emphasis is shifted to discuss caring for these clients on a daily basis—the other 362 days of the year when they aren't hospitalized.

Joe's Story

For several years before we revised our curriculum, Colleen taught clinicals at the local veteran's hospital (VA). She loved the VA and everything about it. The clients were not only interesting but also very eager and willing to work with student nurses. One day, a student was preparing to discharge Joe, a gentleman admitted with severe congestive heart failure. Over the course of his 5-day hospitalization, the doctors and nurses successfully diuresed 52 pounds off Joe. As part of his discharge teaching, the student remembered what she learned in class about the importance of monitoring daily weights as a reflection of fluid volume status. She thought this would be important information to discuss with Joe prior to discharge. The student was more than disillusioned when Joe said that not only did he not have a scale but he also had no money, or interest, in purchasing one. The idea of daily weights was simply out of the question, never mind the fact that Joe did not have a stable place to live and spent most of his days eating and sleeping at the local bar.

In discussing this issue with Colleen in the hallway, the student reviewed what else she learned in lecture regarding the symptom experience of heart failure. With some help, she did recall hearing that although there are well over two dozen different symptoms of heart failure each individual consistently experiences his own symptoms in the exact same order during each episode of heart failure. Yes, there was the clue! The student and Colleen went back to talk with Joe about what had been happening prior to his admission. He discussed how over a period of several weeks, he noticed having to move his belt notch over several spaces, allowing for more room. "In fact," he recalled, "by the time I came here, I had moved my belt over 5 notches." That's about 10 pounds per notch. The student and Colleen worked out with Joe that he would call the VA the next time he noticed that he had to move his belt one notch over from where it was at the time of discharge. He thought that made good sense. That wasn't exactly "by the book" but close enough.

We love the above teaching episode because it challenges instructors and students to question the nature of the content taught as well as the hidden assumptions that underlie it. Clearly monitoring fluid volume status is an important strategy for managing heart failure, probably one of the most important interventions a nurse could teach a client to continue at home. However, it's the way we present this information that could potentially backfire with our students. Check any medical-surgical textbook and review the interventions for congestive heart failure. Undoubtedly, daily weights are often regarded as the gold standard for monitoring fluid volume status. Admit a client to the acute-care unit and daily weights will most assuredly be part of the nursing-care plan, and acute-care nurses will dutifully weigh their patients at 6:00 every morning. But what happens when a student encounters a client like Joe? Students and nurses alike become mentally immobile when they encounter the Joes of the world. Clients are negatively portrayed as "noncompliant" or "unwilling" to participate in their care.

What are we teaching in cases such as Joe's, and what assumptions are we making? Sometimes it's the unconscious message, the unspoken words that come across so poignantly—the subtle facial expressions or the sigh of impatience communicates to a student that Joe has stretched us to our limits.

Because most textbooks focus on the nurse's role in managing illnesses in an acute care setting, emphasis is placed on those interventions a nurse would expect to perform in that setting, such as daily weights, monitoring vital signs, and so on. Given the highly structured setting of acute care and clear lines of authority, little, if any, consideration is given to alternative interventions if a patient refuses. In addition, textbooks present copious amounts of information clients must learn in order to manage at home. The assumption being that the nurse will transfer his or her monitoring duties to either the client or a family member (if there is one) who will happily continue to perform these responsibilities post-discharge.

What else are we teaching? We're inadvertently teaching a gamut of reactions we don't intend to convey—rigidity, inflexibility, lack of creativity, intolerance, and paternalism, to name a few. We also assume that the interventions students read about in their textbooks are doable for all our clients. Isn't this a bit presumptuous? Little, if any, discussion addresses the Joes of the world. If it does, the conversation most often centers on how to persuade Joe into weighing himself everyday. Frequently, this type of monologue is referred to as "patient education." As nursing educators, we handicap our students if we don't proceed beyond where the usual nursing text leaves off and help them understand that true learning, whether in an academic or therapeutic relationship, arises out of dialogue between the nurse and the client.

Viewing chronic illness through the lenses of self-regulation, caregiver concerns, and stigma helps us to engage our students in problematizing commonplace assumptions. By making what is familiar strange, we teach a strategy for disrupting existing power relations and thus promote development of nurses who can enact the college's values of justice, truth, compassion, partnership, and community. Such critical thinking is essential if our students are to become effective client advocates, a role they will need to play regardless of the setting in which they practice. Many of our graduates will initially work in acute-care settings. Presenting nursing care of individuals with chronic health problems in the context of living a life enhances their appreciation for what clients with either acute illness or exacerbations of chronic conditions face upon discharge. The focus on tertiary prevention in the theory course emphasizes nursing management outside the hospital and provides students with valuable information about preparing clients for their return home, or in an increasing number of instances, to shelters or the street.

We are continually challenged by the daunting task of synthesizing all the content in a manner that allows students to learn the difference between physiological, psychological, social, and spiritual care while keeping at the forefront the holistic nature of health. Originally, the course was divided into three distinct units, with the course concepts of self-regulation, stigma, and caregiver issues each representing a unit. We would then try to select which topics best represented the concept. For certain topics, this wasn't too difficult. For example, HIV/AIDS content was discussed under the concept of stigma. Diabetes was discussed under self-regulation. Other topics, however, weren't quite so clear. Take liver disease—does it best fit with stigma (given that a great deal of liver disease is alcohol related), or is self-regulation a better fit? What about caregivers—aren't they often impacted by family members living with liver disease?

Clearly, the entire notion of fitting content areas into categories was absurd, and the process itself negated the idea of whole person care. At best, these themes needed to be introduced at the beginning of the semester and then integrated throughout the rest of the semester. Currently, our first class session is spent, in part, discussing the course themes by reading the personal narratives presented in chapter 3.

Generally speaking, medical-surgical content is taught in the first class period of the week (Monday), and the mental health content is taught during the second class of the week (Friday). Colleen has greater expertise and experience in medical-surgical nursing, and Pamela has greater authority as regards psychiatric nursing. Hypothetically, Colleen is accountable for the pathophysiological content and care of the client requiring medical surgical nursing care, while psychopathology and psychosocial-spiritual care is Pamela's responsibility. In actuality this separation is artificial and made to simplify the topics for the students. In our experience, it is the rare client who has a discrete illness and whose response to his/her illness is not manifested in all four dimensions of health. Our whole-person care frame dictates that we both attend to physical, mental, social, and spiritual aspects of any of the topics we teach.

We strive to instill in our students the ability to provide whole person care for individuals and families experiencing chronic illness and to promote the social change necessary to allow such care. Though continually teased by the temptation to simply tell our students everything we think they need to know toward that end, we have come to understand that "Education dominated by preconceived images of what must be learned can hardly be educational. Authentic teaching and learning requires a live encounter with the unexpected, an element of suspense and surprise, an evocation of that which we did not know until it happened" (Palmer, 1990, p. 76). The course objectives guide what we hope to teach each semester, but it is only when we are able to engage our students in active dialogue that they learn what they need to know to become competent, caring practitioners.

What is distinctive about the chronic illness theory course is the *storied approach* to teaching about nursing care in chronic illness that was introduced in chapter 3. It is our particular version of what has in the last decade come to be generically referred to as narrative pedagogy. People by nature lead storied lives and tell stories of those lives (Clandinin & Connelly, 1994). Stories have value in the clinical arena because they "often convey the essence of a particular event or period of time in one's individual or family history" and thus "are critical sources of information about etiology, diagnosis, treatment and prognosis from the patient's point of view" (Nagai-Jacobson & Burkhardt, 1996, p. 54). In the educational setting the pedagogical value of stories, or anecdotal narratives, lies in their ability to capture student attention, involve them personally, transform them, and measure their interpretive sense (Van Manen, 1990). Because we dream and daydream, remember, anticipate, hope, despair, believe, doubt, plan, revise, criticize, construct, gossip, learn, hate, and love by narrative, stories provide a natural and familiar form of explanation for students and thus facilitates their involvement in learning (Hardy, 1977, cited in Gere, Fairbanks, Howes, Roop, Schaafsma, 1992, p. 150).

A STORIED APPROACH

Our storied approach to whole person care is predicated on the belief that nursing is essentially an interpersonal process concerned with humans and their relationships with themselves and their environments and how these affect their health and well being. Understanding the story of those facing chronic illness figures prominently in the nurse's ability to intervene therapeutically. So, too, does the nurse's understanding of his/her own story. We share stories that blend objective and subjective knowing about chronic illness to foster a narrative aptitude in our students and enhance their capacity to reflect on the meaning of that experience and their reactions to it. What follows are descriptions of a number of types of stories, or narrative strategies, we have found quintessential in helping our students grasp essential nursing science and understand the lived experience of individuals and families coping with chronic illness.

Grand Narratives in the Empiric Mode

Our storied approach does not preclude lecturing, and in reality many class periods include a segment in which one of us, or a guest speaker, relays information in a conventional didactic format. We live in the *real* (i.e., material) world and thus cannot escape the need to convey concrete, factual material in our course. Assuring that our students become adept nurses requires that "It depends" perpetually modify the *facts* we teach though. Every time we convey absolute information, we do as Vella suggests and invite our students to "question, argue, and edit in light of their own life experience" (2002, p. 174).

We do relay scientific knowledge as it is portrayed in the current academic and professional literature, but we encourage our students to challenge the tentativeness of what we know, no matter how passionately we convey it. Interwoven with discussion of nursing care in chronic illness is exploration of how the knowledge we are assuming is constructed. Much of what we now presume was once controversial, and the things we most take for granted are the very ones we most need to question. Whatever seems natural, obvious, self-evident, or universal actually has a history, a reason for being the way that it is. That reason, and the subsequent effects of "the way things are" can reveal much about a given society's power structure. Those things we come to take for granted embody particular values by determining what is or is not normal.

Setting the Tone Stories

The invitation, let alone the expectation, that students critique or challenge their professors' thinking of can be an intimating for both parties. A free exchange of ideas, feelings, and ways of doing things is contingent on a safe milieu. We regularly assert that confidentiality is just as essential in the classroom as it is in the clinical setting. So, too, are a nonjudgmental attitude and openness to diversity. At the most basic level, we move our students into a narrative frame by expressing interest in them, listening when they do speak up, and applauding when they have the courage to ask questions.

We really do care what our students do and do not understand about the experience of chronic illness. Sometimes to get them to reveal their uncertainties we have to prime the pump by revealing ways in which we are fallible. Colleen loves to tell about the time when we were introduced to the portable defibrillator during our last CPR recertification. After verbally walking though the procedure for its proper use in a cardiac arrest and practicing several times, Pamela felt confident enough to have the instructor evaluate our abilities. We preformed brilliantly, right up to the point where Pamela, after conscientiously checking that Colleen was clear of the device so that the shock could be safely delivered to the fictitious victim, enthusiastically hit the wrong button and turned the defibrillator off! Though we require students to be prepared and function in class and clinical in a competent manner, we want them to know mistakes are inevitable, seldom irreparable when owned up to, and often promote significant learning.

Sometimes we offer a narrative as a means of elucidating more ephemeral concepts, such as spiritual care. Stories can also convey an acceptance that there are times when even an experienced practitioner doesn't know what to do. And, they can underscore that nursing intervention in chronic illness often needs to take the form of being with, rather than doing to, the client. Such was the case one semester several years ago when Pamela supervised a group of students on the inpatient psychiatric unit at our local VA hospital.

A Moment of Grace

One semester, a fellow well known to the staff was readmitted to the unit in a decompensated state after having been in the community for about a year. His extreme agitation fueled their fear that, as with multiple previous admissions, he would become a "disposition problem" and they would be stuck trying to manage the milieu, which would inevitably escalate in response to his persistent and unremitting psychosis. When everyone predicted it would be months before he would settle down and a suitable placement would be found, I judged them harshly for setting up a self-fulfilling prophecy. After several weeks, I had an opportunity to walk in their shoes and was humbled by the challenge they faced daily, hourly, and moment-to-moment.

Though one could see some signs of improvement, the fellow continued to be irritable and had regular outbursts each day. He would wander the unit mumbling, usually incoherently, and occasionally would intrude on the physical space of others or threaten them directly with a closed fist. His shabby appearance revealed an inability to attend to his personal hygiene or to cooperate enough to allow others to assist him.

One morning, I happened on him in the dinning room, sitting all alone. Breakfast was over, and all the other patients had moved into the dayroom or left for their various appointments. Though the patients tended to be very tolerant of one another's shortcomings, their patience for his contentious ramblings was waning. The nurses left him in the dining room, both to give the other patients respite and because they hoped the lesser stimuli there would calm him. Not wanting to leave him all alone, they parked him in front of an old time comic video, thinking it might somehow hold his attention. They were too busy to stay with him, but checked in periodically.

Having progressed to a point where they required little of me, my students were all off attending to the needs of their assigned patients. I alone had the time to sit with this distraught fellow. During his best periods, he muttered quietly to himself. This was punctuated by frantic, nonsensical outbursts, though at several points I could make out an utterance like "No, no! Let the boy have the food. He's starving." Knowing that he was a World War II veteran, I surmised that he was somewhere in Europe reexperiencing the trauma of war. His suffering was palpable. Occasionally he looked at me in a rather menacing manner, and I had to steady myself to remain with him. I don't know if I was trying to reassure him or myself as I periodically told him very softly, "You are safe here."

When he would appear to notice the video, I would ask him about the characters. Mostly he responded with gibberish but several times surprised me with a laugh. He would momentarily connect with the characters on the screen, calling them by name. After each name, I would whisper, "That's right." He would then turn, and though he didn't really relate to me, I felt some acknowledgment of my presence. I continued to sit with him. Though I had the time to do so, I didn't have a clue what I was doing.

He tired of the video and began to walk around. As his movement increased, so did his agitation. He headed toward the dayroom, barking orders at some unseen marauders. I tensed with a sense of obligation to calm him and protect the other patients. I gently encouraged him to take a seat. Much to my amazement, he complied. He perched on a chair at the periphery of the dayroom. I pulled another close to continue my vigil. His shouts softened a bit, and he teared up. "No, no! Let the boy eat first! He is starving." He grasped his head in his hands and shook it back and forth. "No, no, no. Let the boy have it." Now he was sobbing. I wished to comfort him, but I didn't know how. I just sat there while his weeping escalated to loud, mournful wails.

Noticing his distress, one of the nurses brought him some medication. At first the offer of the drug annoyed him, but the nurse said it would help. Was it with resignation, hope or some other emotion that he took it? I couldn't tell, but I knew the relief it might provide would not arrive immediately or be permanent. Having a little more time before my students would return, I continued to sit with him. The momentary lull afforded by his swallowing was broken when he recommenced his lamentation. Witnessing his deep despair began to take its toll. Not knowing how much longer I could bear it, I turned inward. Silently I pleaded for divine intervention. "Please do not let him suffer any more than he can bear!" I felt my eyes filling with tears.

He turned to me fully and said definitively and exceptionally clearly, "What you are doing is helping." We sat in silence together for a few minutes. My students returned to the unit, and to my awareness. Now they needed me more than he did. I thanked him for sitting with me, and excused myself. The rest of my day was draped with tremendous gratitude for having shared a moment of grace.

We view teaching and learning as sacred activities. Ideally, the content in the classroom is shaped by clinical and personal experiences of both faculty and students.

STUDENT STORIES

Even when presenting in a didactic mode, we continually integrate theoretical content with stories from our own lives and practice. We invite students to share their stories to the extent that they are able. We encourage them to discuss how they are applying what they are learning in the theory course to clinical situations in their chronic illness clinical course, and how interactions with real clients in the clinical course shapes their understanding of the more abstract concepts in the theory course.

An assignment, in which we have students write a series of three brief accounts of their own experience with chronic illness allows us to get to know them and to discern their grasp of course concepts at the beginning, middle, and end of the course. We never cease to be amazed by how candid our students are, and reading about the adversity some of them have faced in their personal lives helps put the student experience in perspective and humbles us.

The Wrath of Fibromyalgia

Before I started nursing school, I didn't know what fibromyalgia was, nor did I really care. I didn't even know what it meant when people said they had a chronic illness. I just got really irritated hearing her complain all the time about how tired she was always feeling or about her aches and pains. She wasn't any fun, and I sure couldn't rely on her to come to any of my sporting or other important events at school.

You are probably wondering whom I am talking about right now. Well, it's my mother, who has been burdened with fibromyaligia for the last 10 years.

I look back on my behavior now and I am ashamed of myself. For God's sake, this is my mother I am talking about. I love her but I kept looking at how this illness affected me, and not how it was ripping the life out of her. Something that I didn't realize before was that this illness dropped my mother into a deep depression for the first 5 years after her diagnosis. I just felt like she didn't want to be a part of my life. I couldn't understand that the illness was holding her back.

My mother's fibromyalgia caused severe muscle tension in her upper body, especially her neck and back. That caused her to get migraines that put her out of commission for at least a day. My mother was able to develop a dialectical self where she could feel tingling in her upper back and neck signaling the onset of an attack. Then she would be able to take it easy, and with the proper medicine, the effects would be lessened. She would also get lower flank pain that would prevent her from even walking. She still takes muscle relaxants, and for a while she also took antidepressants. Before nursing school, I couldn't understand the full impact of side effects from these drugs. They knocked her out, and she would be asleep more than she was awake. Sometimes she'd skip the medicine, even though she knew it would help, because she didn't want to spend the whole day in bed. She always had to weigh the pros and cons.

I understand now that having good days, and bad days are part and parcel of chronic illness. On bad days, Mom slips into the illness routine, though, and it is hard for my family to understand that this is worse for her than it is for us. She'll stay in bed all day because that's easier than dealing with the physical, emotional, and mental pain. Like any chronic illness, fribromyalgia is an energy drainer.

I am happy that the disease hasn't had any direct effect on her cognition and that she can pursue her goal of becoming a social worker. I am so proud of her. She takes a couple of classes each semester and is actually scheduled to finish at the same time I'll be graduating. She works hard, even though she doesn't feel well, but she does get down on herself when she only gets a B or has to miss a class because of a migraine. She has no idea how proud her family is of her for pursuing an education when she is burdened with a chronic illness.

My mom also tries to get help for herself by attending support groups. I can say that I am much more supportive and understanding than I was before I got into nursing school, but I have no idea what it feels like to have fibromyalgia. I think that it is really good for her to vent her frustrations with people who understand where she's coming from. She has a lot of anger related to her illness. She really doesn't feel it's fair and is frustrated that there is no cure. She struggles as well with having to convince others she even has a disease. I worry what she'll do if she hears one more time that it's all in her head.

I think that if I had to walk a day in the shoes of someone who is chronically ill I would do a 180. I don't want to face that I am not invincible, and I don't want to have to depend on others to complete activities of daily living. Every time I do patient care now, I think about this in the hope that I might become the kind of nurse who can make a difference in the life of someone who suffers like my mom.

We urge students to pay attention to their clients, to notice with an open heart and mind what is going on with them, inside and out. We take the same stance with the students, in as much as how they are doing impacts on learning about nursing care in chronic illness. Clients and students cannot or will not always share the depth of their experience, though, and it is not possible or necessarily advantageous to know everything about each one. At times, fragile students reveal more than they intended, or their peers wanted to know, about their own personal battles with chronic illness.

Like clients, students sometimes share too much information—TMI, as we lovingly refer to that particular phenomenon—and can flood the classroom, inappropriately divert student attention, and impede learning. Many of the topics explored in class evoke strong emotional responses that can catch students by surprise, lower their defenses, stir up unresolved issues, and leave them feeling quite vulnerable. We have to be constantly attentive to the affective tone in our classroom, reign in those students whose urgency to voice their experiences impinges on others, and make space for the more introverted members to share if they wish. As faculty, our responsibility extends beyond the 2 hours of each class period, and we make ourselves available to help students contain any concerns that arise in response to the course material, or to refer them to others who can help them to do so.

CASE STUDIES: PUTTING PATHOPHYSIOLOGY IN THE CONTEXT OF A WHOLE PERSON

Before the advent of the chronic illness classes, the "liver content" in the Edgewood nursing curriculum was covered in a traditional medical-surgical nursing course. The colleague who was responsible for the course asked Colleen to present the topic, because she had much experience working with individuals whose health was compromised by liver disease. As was often the case, she began her preparation by reading the chapter in the course textbook, taking notes on the content she felt was particularly important. As a fairly experienced lecturer, her intent was to present the standard lecture on liver failure, that is, review physiology, discuss pathophysiology, and identify nursing care issues using the nursing process as the basic format. Before she had completed her first page of notes, she was already disengaged. Wondering how she could make the material remotely interesting, she reflected on how she had learned about liver disease. That led her to write the following case study as the format for the lecture and discussion.

Although the case study focuses on an acute care experience, it tells the true story of a man named Ben. Imagine how difficult it must be for students attempting to understand the complexities of liver failure, having never even seen someone with the disease. Ben's story imparts the reality of someone trying to live a life with a deadly disease, and provides students the opportunity to comprehend a different perspective while applying nursing knowledge. Interspersed with Ben's story are Colleen's notes that segue into class discussion about the *realities* of providing care for someone as unique as him. The clinical discussion topics are presented in bold type.

Ben: Living a Life With Liver Disease

I'll never forget Ben. I was a student at the VA when I first encountered him. He was living with advanced cirrhosis and would require frequent hospital admissions to manage the numerous medical problems that kept coming up. It seems that on this particular day, Ben had consumed a large quantity of beans and other sources of protein in the hospital cafeteria and literally passed out in his bowl of bean soup. He was admitted to the medical floor, comatose. His medical diagnosis was hepatic encephalopathy. The medical goal was to decrease his serum ammonia levels. This was when I first met Ben.

Ben was a nursing instructor's dream comes true. What instructor doesn't enjoy challenging his or her students with the complex pathophysiology of liver failure? I can hear her now. Why does he have ascites, why is he on a protein restricted diet, why is he hypoglycemic, why is he receiving spironolactone and not lasix, why is he getting lactulose, and why is he bleeding—why, why, why, why? Where do I start? All that seems so medical. Sure, I needed to know all that, but let's look at Ben first. Who is this guy?

Ben was in his late 60s. He was by all intents and purposes a bum, a street person. His wife had died several years ago, and he had no children or any other relatives. He was literally alone. I don't know the circumstances surrounding Ben's alcohol consumption, it really seems rather unimportant at this point, but he has a past and present history of consuming large quantities of alcohol. Does it really matter if it's brandy or gin? Ben was an engineer in his other life, but is seems, somehow, things just got away from him. He lives in a flophouse on the city's south side. Occasionally, his landlady would offer him a meal.

Clinical Day 1

Ben was comatose. His ammonia level was over 100 (normal is 30–70 µg/dl). He was receiving lactulose, folic acid, vitamin K+, and thiamine. I distinctly remember the lactulose. It comes in a thick sticky liquid and was given down his nasogastric tube. It causes unbelievable diarrhea. Everyone seemed to think that was great, except for me. I had to clean it all up. Ben was rather apple shaped, with a large ascitic abdomen and no body fat. His coccyx was rapidly becoming excoriated because of his diarrhea. That was my first day.

Discussion
Medications
Ascites
Nursing Care

Clinical Day 2

Regardless of his situation, Ben was a likeable guy. He was totally disrespectful of doctors and nurses. "You can all go to hell" were his first words when he awoke. I was surprised to see the rapid recovery in just 2 days. Ben was awake, appropriate (most of the time), and eating. Forty-eight hours of lactulose every 6 hours had decreased his NH3 to 40. It was sad to see how alcohol had destroyed his body. On rounds, the residents asked him to perform various neurological tests: touch hand to nose, stretch arms out in front with eyes closed, and so on. Ben performed them all poorly. Once outside the room, the residents laughed at him. It hurt. The progress notes said Wernicke-Korsakof syndrome, asterixis, and so on. It didn't sound good. Ben had been placed on a low protein/low sodium diet, with a 1,500 cc fluid limit. He ate everything place in front of him and then went to the cafeteria and ate more! Eggs were his favorite. He drank water out of the fountains with no regard for his fluid limit. His doctors would yell at the nurses because he kept gaining weight. Ben weighed 155 pounds, most of it ascites fluid. His dry weight was probably 140. To solve the water problem, the residents had the water shut off in his room. Ben didn't seem to mind; he'd had a hard life, and he could get all the water he wanted down the hall or in the cafeteria. It was more of a problem for the nurses not having water in his room than it was for Ben.

Discussion
Diet therapy
Neurological impairments
Management strategies

Clinical Day 3

Ben's potassium had been rising. It was now up to 6.1 mEq. On rounds, the doctors were discussing diuretic management. Ben had been on spironolactone (aldactone) as a diuretic. It was thought that this was the most likely cause of his increased K+. They decided to stop his spironolactone and to try diuresing Ben with lasix. While this bedside conversation was occurring, Ben kept asking about going home. He could care less about what his potassium level was. He just wanted to leave. I kept wondering what that meant for a homeless person. He really didn't have a home. Ben's room didn't have the usual assortment of cards, gifts, or flowers. No one came to visit. I doubt that anyone even knew he was in the hospital. Would his room still be there or would the landlady give it to someone else? I made a mental note to check into this. What an odd feeling. Ben had managed to befriend several of the other patients, though. It was not uncommon to see them laughing together while watching TV in the dayroom at the end of the hall or even engaging in a rousing game of cards. Too bad he was so sick, but, you know, it didn't seem to matter to him. Life had a different meaning for him. His hematocrit had started to drop. Although it was never very high to begin with, usually around 33%, it was now down to 25%. His doctors suspected bleeding. The most likely source was from his esophageal varices. They were discussing treatment options amongst themselves. Funny, no one ever asked Ben what he wanted done if he had a huge bleed. Because of his neurological damage, they felt he was incompetent.

Discussion
Role of aldosterone
Portal hypertension: management options
Meaning of illness to person

Clinical Day 4

Ben wasn't in his room when I arrived. He had been transferred to the medical ICU during the night. He had gone into hepatorenal syndrome. I didn't understand what the kidneys had to do with liver failure, but somehow his kidneys had suddenly decided to fail. I was told that hepatorenal syndrome is untreatable. It's usually at this point that medicine throws in the towel; there is nothing more to offer. "Offer"—what an interesting notion. What exactly was it that we offered Ben? We shut off his water, nagged him about everything he ate, and periodically stuck needles in his arm. He, in turn, obliged us with a toothless grin. Now we offer him death. He died shortly after his arrival in ICU. I didn't quite understand why he was transferred to the ICU to begin with. Can't people die in their rooms? My nursing instructor said it was a good learning experience. I guess it must have been because I still remember Ben 25 years after his death. During my nursing career, I have since seen dozens of Bens; I've given large quantities of lactulose and transfused more esophageal bleeders than I care to remember, but I can't forget Ben. Today, we transplant people like Ben. I wonder what he would have done if this had been an option 25 years ago?

Discussion
Renal failure
Caring and curing

After writing about Ben, Colleen found that preparing material for theory classes became easier and more interesting to the students and to her. Students preferred stories about people to the standard lecture format. She wrote about Glenn—a farmer with an eighth grade education trying to manage his expensive, complex, and ever changing medical regimen for severe hypertension; Candy—a nursing student with rheumatoid arthritis; Dickey—a cheese maker turned truck driver living with diabetes; and Uncle Lee—who died from emphysema. (These cases can be found in Appendix A.)

Colleen's stories serve as the basis for classroom discussion. Students receive written copies of the cases to help them prepare prior to class and to use for the purposes of note taking in class. Students bring in their experiences with clients from clinical and also converse about other people they know who are living with chronic illness and experiencing similar situations. This format simultaneously fulfills two functions. It provides students the opportunity to study nursing content in an applied context, which aids retention. It also offers students the chance to gain knowledge about integrating nursing care according to the individual/family needs—the art of nursing science. Studying how to implement sound scientific knowledge becomes equally important as learning the facts. This helps ward off potential paralysis the first time students encounter a client similar to Ben or Joe.

Differentiating acute care interventions from the issues faced by clients on a daily basis as they live their lives with chronic illness is of paramount importance. The cases emphasize how to recognize trouble as well as self-regulatory strategies that promote partnerships in care. Integrating the three primary concepts of the course—self-regulation, stigma, and caregiver issues—becomes effortless in the context of case stories.

Unfortunately, it does not take students long to become discouraged by clients who, despite all the well-intended actions on the part of the students, don't change their actions. Students find it exceptionally difficult to understand that education does not necessarily change behavior. Undergraduates idealistically believe that clearly what's needed is *more* and *better* patient education. Using lived experiences as didactic content allows students to appreciate the reality of our (the nurse's) expectations as these come into conflict with the client's reality. Several models, such as the Health Belief Model, conceptualize the complexities of health behavior. For novice nursing students, models appear too abstract and are oftentimes difficult to apply, but students do understand this very simple equation:

Values + Beliefs = Behavior

When we discuss a nurse trying to get a teenager to quit smoking, we're attempting to change a behavior. That can't happen very easily without understanding the values and beliefs involved. Adolescents' values, as a result of peer pressure, include the desire to be a part of the in group or to be cool. In the adolescent belief system is the notion that they are immortal—"Everyone else will get cancer but not me"—or "I'm in control, I can quit anytime." Adding the value of being cool to the belief of control and immortality allows them the behavior of smoking. Understanding and addressing the values and beliefs will change how a nurse approaches this issue. This simple equation helps students revisit the nursing process and assess their clients more thoroughly. It also suggests that nurses should know their clients as people before attempting to implement actions aimed at changing behaviors.

This equation is frequently referred to throughout the course during our discussions/lectures in class. Students gain an appreciation for why someone's blood pressure is out of control despite an aggressive medical regimen prescribed. *Reason:* The client had to share his medication with his wife. Or why someone consistently gains 10 lbs between dialysis treatments. *Reason:* The client can only afford canned soup and baloney sandwiches for lunch and dinner. Understanding more than the disease and the appropriate textbook interventions is essential in learning to provide whole-person care.

Once students understand the importance of knowing their clients' values and beliefs, learning to respect them becomes another hurdle. It is difficult to respect someone's belief that vinegar and honey is a better antihypertensive agent than a beta-blocker, or the depression era mindset wherein frugality is so highly valued that clients cut their nitro patches in half to save money, or clients who never take prophylactic medication because it is far too wasteful. Students come to accept that maybe, just maybe, their clients are doing the best that they can, given their values, beliefs, economic status, and level of education. Despite these challenges, students learn to separate the person from their actions and to become much more grounded and realistic in the expectations they have for their clients.

Reviewing Ben's story and the sample cases in Appendix A makes it readily apparent that not everything is covered in the scenarios presented. However, it is through the stories that students realize the content areas they should revisit and need to master to adequately develop their knowledge of the topic. Stories are not intended to *cover* everything. Our stories provide examples of how we let go of content. They represent a scholarly assessment of what information students might use as a foundation upon which to further build their nursing knowledge base. As such, stories offer realistic alternatives that blend didactic content with practical application for clinical practice. Realizing that classroom instructors will never be able to cover everything, letting go of content provides a new approach that enriches classroom content and ultimately enhances critical thinking. While we let go of content, we teach our students the skills necessary to find the factual information needed, to fill in the blanks of their knowledge base, to analyze what is appropriate for each individual clients' situation, and to evaluate the outcome.

STORIES TO PUT MENTAL ILLNESS IN ITS PLACE

Pamela has primary responsibility for presenting course content related to the care of individuals and families dealing with mental illness and addressing the psychosocial-spiritual sequela of chronic illness in general. In addition to acquainting students with the nuances of providing nursing care for persons labeled with the various psychiatric diagnoses evident in the topic list in Table 4.1, she is charged with helping students examine preconceived prejudicial ideas they have about people who have psychological impairments. Metaphorically, this necessitates having ready access to the stigma lens for each class period.

Being clear about one's boundaries as a caregiver is essential for survival in nursing. It is especially apropos and challenging when dealing with mentally ill clients. Their characterology and symptomatology can lead them to transgress accepted social norms or render them vulnerable when the caregiver is not clear about the nature of the relationship. Developing the therapeutic use of self in our students is contingent on recognition of their own strengths and limits. Only then can they avoid projecting their issues on the clients or personalizing client reactions that really have nothing to do with them. In the clinical class, students are positioned to actually provide care that much of this learning gets enacted, but in some regards, the theory class serves as launching pad for that experience. Although the clients' students work with in the psychosocial-spiritual component of the clinical course, it is nowhere near as scary or dangerous as they fantasize, although some clients do present with problematic behaviors that can impinge on safety. The theory course provides a less threatening environment, one in which students can grapple with their fears and explore some of the interpersonal skills and techniques necessary for intervening with clients whose worlds may be intellectually, emotionally, socially, and/or spiritually tenuous.

Like Colleen, though to a more limited degree, Pamela intersperses her classroom teaching with cases fashioned from clinical practice. To give students a more vicarious understanding of the experience of chronic mental illness and issues at the end of life from both the client and caregiver perspective, she employs four other kinds of stories as well. The first of these could be called *cases al la mode*—synopses of current events reported in the popular media. Classroom discussions regularly take a turn toward pondering whether those involved in recent local or national crimes might meet the criteria for a given mental illness. We query as well how the prevalence of war and other violence, social inequities, and the general pace of life might figure in the development of psychiatric symptoms and the construction of certain diagnostic categories. Descriptions of the three other types of stories follow.

Literary Cases

The second type of tale Pamela employs arises from popular and professional literature. Reading *Gracefully Insane*, Alex Beam's (2001) best selling portrait of McLean Hospital, one of America's oldest psychiatric institutions, gives students a historical perspective on mental health care in this country. Amusing anecdotes about some of its famous and infamous patients captures their interest and draws them into factual descriptions of somatic and interpersonal therapies. Personal accounts of encounters with chronic illness like *Tuesdays With Morrie*, Mitch Albom's reminiscence of the time he spent with his cherished dying professor Morrie Schwartz, and Pat Deegan's exceedingly poignant story of reclaiming her sense of value in the face of being labeled with chronic schizophrenia are other examples of stories used in class. Both illustrate the notion of self-regulation. Albom's tale also enhances student empathy for family and friends taking on the caregiver role. Deegan's decree that "It is important to understand that we are faced with recovering not just from mental illness, but also from the effect of being labeled mentally ill" (p. 10, 1993) reiterated throughout the course highlights the extent of stigmatization of mental illness.

Video Cases

A third and frequently employed story form is that of video, both educational and popular. Table 4.2 provides a listing of currently used videos and the course topics each elucidates. Most of the videos are viewed in advance and, along with assigned readings, are intended to prepare students for class lecture, discussion and experiential activities. A few of the videos, as indicated in Table 4.2, are shown in class and serve as a more academic counterpoint to Hollywood's rendition of the various disorders.

Pamela makes available online optional worksheets that students may use to assess whether they have grasped essential concepts from the readings and videos. Her PowerPoint lecture notes, accessible online, double as worksheet answer keys. Each topic area has associated "critical questions" that help ready students for class, and give them an opportunity to earn points toward their final grade. The questions call for reasoned judgment and have no definitive answers, though points may be deducted if answers are incomplete or inaccurate.

A brief overview of the class period devoted to "Nursing Care of the Client with Psychosis: Case Example—Schizophrenia" helps illustrate how the readings, videos, worksheets, and critical questions are used in the psychosocial-spiritual component of NR3340. As preparation, the students read a chapter in a psychiatric nursing text that describes relevant DSM-IV and nursing diagnoses, presents hypothesized etiologies, and explores a variety of treatment strategies and nursing interventions. Many students will then complete the associated worksheet to test their comprehension. Next they view *A Beautiful Mind,* a popular movie that takes a number of liberties in portraying the mathematician and Nobel Prize winner John Nash's struggle with schizophrenia. It does, however, illustrate the trajectory and symptomology of the disorder, as well as some of its interpersonal and social ramifications. Afterwards, the students are ready to grapple with the following critical questions that serve as a springboard for classroom discussion:

1. John Nash was a Nobel prize-winning mathematician who developed a groundbreaking economic theory and struggled with a debilitating thought disorder. Give some examples from the movie, *A Beautiful Mind,* that substantiate that John Nash suffered from both positive and negative symptoms of schizophrenia.
2. Farrell and colleagues note that, "Because the reality distortions of psychosis create a potential risk for agitation or violence, safety

TABLE 4.2 Films and Video Cases You Can Use in Class

Content Topic	Video Case	Critical Questions
Chronic Mental Illness Case Model: Social Construction of Stigma	*Back Wards to Back Streets:* This 1980 video documentary, produced, written, and directed by Roger Weisberg, Public Policy Productions, portrays the plight of many patients who ended up homeless or in inadequate housing subsequent to the Supreme Court decision to deinstitutionalize them. Some examples of successful community mental health treatment programs are also described.	1. Access the National Alliance for the Mentally Ill (NAMI) Web site (http//www.nami.org) and click on their stigma alerts listing. Identify one listing and indicate whether you were surprised, delighted, annoyed (etc.) that NAMI tagged the identified party. 2. Deegan (1993, Recovering our sense of value after being labeled. *Journal of Psychosocial Nursing, 31*(4), 7–11) notes that once you're labeled with a mental illness "everything you do gets understood in reference to your illness" (p. 9). Give an example from your own experience that either supports or negates this stance. 3. After viewing Back Wards to Back Streets, identify several pros and cons of deinstitutionalization.
Psychotic disorders Case Model: schizophrenia	*A Beautiful Mind* 60 Minutes (3/31/02): Mike Wallace interviews John Nash about his life and the movie, *A Beautiful Mind.* This pairing affords an opportunity for students to contrast Hollywood's version of John Nash's life with his own. Students are also given Web sites to explore further.	1. John Nash was a Nobel prize-winning mathematician who developed a groundbreaking economic theory and struggled with a debilitating thought disorder. Give some examples from the movie, *A Beautiful Mind,* that substantiate that John Nash suffered from both positive and negative symptoms of schizophrenia.

(continued)

TABLE 4.2 *(continued)*

Content Topic	Video Case	Critical Questions
		2. Farrell and colleagues note that "because the reality distortions of psychosis create a potential risk for agitation or violence, safety is of paramount importance" (1998, p. 190). They note as well the importance of rapport in working with psychotic individuals (1998, p. 191). What were some of the things that John Nash's family and friends did to decrease his underlying (although sometimes indistinguishable) anxiety?
		3. In what ways does the movie help to overcome and/or reinforce stereotypes about schizophrenia and mental illness in general?
Mood Disorders Case models: depression & mania	*Mr. Jones:* the value of this melodramatic view of bipolar disorder lies in Richard Gere's believable renditions of depression and mania and, ironically, in the implausible romance between him and his therapist. The later phenomenon provides ample fuel for meaningful class discussions about ethical treatment and the boundaries of therapeutic relationships.	1. Identify— a. At least three behaviors Mr. Jones demonstrated in the community that would help support Dr. Bowen's assessment on admission that he has a bipolar affective disorder and was in a manic phase. b. At least two symptoms of depression he evidenced at Howard's house and in the hospital that support a diagnosis of depression.
		2. In completing a mental status exam of Mr. Jones, how would you describe his insight and judgment?

TABLE 4.2 *(continued)*

Content Topic Video Case	Critical Questions
	3. Both Mr. Jones and his friend Howard demonstrated some skill in managing crisis situations. Howard was successful in getting Mr. Jones out of precarious circumstances on the roof. Mr. Jones saved Dr. Bowen's life by intervening when Mr. Altman assaulted her. Identify at least two things each man did that enhanced the likelihood of a positive outcome.
Safety Concerns Case Model: Restraints and seclusion — Replays of relevant clips from *A Beautiful Mind* and *Mr. Jones* that depict points at which each of the main characters poses a threat to himself or others are shown in class.	
Iatrogenic Disease Case Model: psychopharmacology — Screening for tardive dyskinesia video shown in class.	
Substance-Related Disorders Case Model: multiple substance abuse — *28 Days*	
Anxiety Disorders Case Model: ODC — *As Good As It Gets*	1. In what ways does Melvin fit DSM-IV-TR criteria for obsessive-compulsive disorder? 2. One of the main themes of NRS 340 is how the experience of chronic illness challenges self-regulation. How did Melvin's various symptoms (i.e., behavioral quirks) enhance his sense of control and how did they detract from it?

(continued)

TABLE 4.2   *(continued)*

Content Topic	Video Case	Critical Questions
		3. Suppose Melvin needed to be hospitalized on an acute medical-surgical unit following a hernia repair. What advice would you give the nursing staff providing his care to help prevent exacerbation of his psychiatric symptoms and facilitate his recovery?
Personality Disorders Case Models: obsessive-compulsive, narcissistic, borderline antisocial personalities	*Girl, Interrupted* Personality disorders video shown in class	
Dissociative Disorders Case Models: PTSD and DID	*Prince of Tides*	
Eating Disorders Case Models: anorexia, bulimia, and obesity	*Dying to Be Thin* shown in class. Originally broadcast 12/12/02 on PBS's Nova, the video presents stories of sometimes life-threatening eating disorders, particularly anorexia and bulimia. *http://www.pbs.org/wgbh/nova/thin/*	1. Self-regulation: Although binge-eating disorder has been proposed for inclusion in the next version of the DSM, obesity is not a mental illness. What, if any, impact do you think legitimizing binge-eating as a medical label might have on the incidence of obesity in this country? 2. Caregiver Concerns: After completing assigned readings, briefly discuss what you would do if you noted any of the early signs or health consequences in a friend or family member. What are some of the things that help you or keep you from addressing a possible eating disorder in someone you care about?

TABLE 4.2 *(continued)*

Content Topic	Video Case	Critical Questions
		3. Stigma: After completing assigned readings, respond to the following question. In what ways do the attitudes apparent in the two articles alleviate or promote stereotypical views of people who are obese?
Mental Disorders of Childhood or Adolescence Case Models: ADHD and autism	*Behavioral Disorders in Children* and *Ordinary People*	1. How does the physician on the *Behavioral Disorders of Children* video who discusses the therapeutic effects of ritalin explain the fact that a chemical stimulant results in a child's achieving more organized, constructive behavior?
		2. What are some of the most important things you've learned about therapeutic relationships this semester that will help you intervene with individuals like the four children in the video and their families?
		3. The video *Ordinary People* was made in 1980. Identify some stigmatized views of mental illness that were depicted in the video and indicate whether they continue to be prevalent today.
		4. Identify a priority nursing diagnosis for each of the three Jarrett family members and one nursing intervention you could use to address it: Conrad: Beth: Calvin:
Facing the End of Life Case Model: professional caregiver concerns	*Wit* *Caring for Mo*—shown in class	

is of paramount importance" (1998, p. 190). They note, as well, that the importance of rapport in working with psychotic individuals (1998, p. 191). What were some of the things that John Nash's family and friends did to decrease his underlying (although sometimes indistinguishable) anxiety?

3. In what ways does the movie help to overcome and/or reinforce stereotypes about schizophrenia and mental illness in general?

The class period begins with a showing of a *60 Minutes* (3/31/00) interview by Mike Wallace with John Nash, his wife, and his younger son Johnny. Pairing this video with *A Beautiful Mind* affords an opportunity for students to contrast Hollywood's version of John Nash's life with his own. Pamela then proceeds to an interactive lecture about schizophrenia and other psychotic disorders from a PowerPoint presentation that includes still shots from *A Beautiful Mind* and links to relevant websites. Students interject with their insights and questions. They have open access to the notes and websites throughout the semester, and those who want to learn more about Nash's life and the most current theories and practices related to schizophrenia can do so at their leisure.

The just described sequence is reenacted in many of the psychosocial-spiritual class sessions. Table 4.2 includes *Critical Questions* used with some of the topic areas and their associated videos. The characters in the videos are like clients the students come to know and understand better over the course of the semester as they learn more about the nature and treatment of mental illness. The fact that some of the video characters are based on the lives of actual people makes them more believable. Susanna Kaysen, like John Nash, is a former McLean patient. The video *Girl, Interrupted,* described in Table 4.2, is based on her book of the same title, which details her almost two year hospitalization there. Students appreciate that in addition to the stories about McLean offered by Beam, Kaysen, and Nash, Pamela has her own story about teaching a psychiatric nursing clinical there in the early 90s.

Caring for individuals with mental illness can be perplexing and demanding, as clients may be rejecting or evoke feelings in the caregiver that interfere with the therapeutic process. Donald Oliver maintains that both technical knowledge and ontological knowing involve concepts, skills, and attitudes, and, thus, effective teaching strategies include cognitive, psychomotor, and affective elements (cited in Vella, 2002, p. 150). The written and video scenarios noted up to this point do evoke visceral responses and provide avenues for exploring possible action and intervention.

Impromptu Stories

Intervening effectively with persons whose mental processes can be manifested in bizarre and sometimes threatening ways requires command of one's own thoughts, feelings, and actions, which requires lots of practice, much of which will be afforded in the clinical course. The fourth story form—dramatization—adds an interactive dimension to classroom cases and gives students a preview of how they might react to inevitable encounters with frustrated, angry, hostile, sad, otherwise emotionally wrought clients in clinical. Occasionally, Pamela has colluded with the college's theatre department or individual students in the course to surprise the rest of class with a topic-relevant client scenario. More often, she intersperses impromptu role playing with the other three types of stories to engage students in challenging situations without actually placing them in harm's way. Integrating neologisms into a lecture on psychosis, periodically striking strange postures, or appearing to attend to internal stimuli give a fuller feeling of what it is like to sit with someone who is actively psychotic. Acting depressed (e.g., evidencing psychomotor retardation or becoming tearful) or manic (e.g., speaking in a rapid, pressured manner and pacing around the classroom) while lecturing about mood disorders not only promotes student attention, it forces them into the story. Shouting at them in the midst of talking about how to manage someone who is angry catches them off guard, just as clients often do.

That such theatrics evoke strong student responses, even when they know it is an act, highlights a fundamental principle in the mental health arena—emotions are contagious! Effective nursing, regardless of the setting or the population being served, requires being able to manage affectively charged situations. Classroom dramatics provide an opportunity to explore how one's thoughts and feelings might lead to action, or immobilization. They are not without some risk though, as Pamela discovered just a few semesters ago when she entered the class period designated as Safety Concerns in a fictitiously bad mood.

Infectious Anxiety

I do not like to admit the relief I felt when that particular group of students graduated. In the year after they moved on from NRS 340 and 341, I would sometimes see a bunch of them together and would reexperience the feelings of immense inadequacy I had the day I violated my cardinal rule, SAFETY FIRST! I espouse that all the time, in the classroom and in clinical settings.

I tell students that a physically and emotionally secure milieu is essential for therapeutic work and learning and that the nurse or teacher has significant responsibility for creating it.

What was I thinking that day? I do vaguely remember feeling uneasy, even before I entered the classroom, but I disregarded the feeling. This was ironic, in light of my continual preaching, "Listen to your gut." I had done this at least 10 times before, and I told myself this was just the usual initial stage fright. I took a deep breath and entered the classroom. I started off being just a little pissy. I didn't offer my usual greetings or really look at anyone. I walked straight to the lectern and kind of slopped my bag down. I rummaged through it as if I couldn't find something quite important. I remember sighing and frowning a lot. As usual, it took a few minutes before anyone seemed to notice. Then, the familiar quizzical looks. Oh yes, she's astute and would pick up right away that I am acting. After all, the schedule says we'll be addressing safety concerns today.

Quickly, it was evident that others are on to me too, and I worry that I will not evoke the tenuousness that facilitates learning. I ratchet it up a level or two. A student comes in late. I shot her a dirty look and shook my head at the rest of the class. She sat down quickly while I launched into "I don't want to hear about parking. I know it stinks. I was here on time." I escalated further, probably pacing around the classroom and getting in the students' space. The exact details are fuzzy now, lost in retrospective shame.

I do remember thinking they all saw me for the phony I was. After talking about anger in an irritable tone I started darting questions at the students. I cut off midsentence those who dared respond, or followed up their comments with massive corrections. I was surprised and pleased when Missy, brave soul, came to the defense of a previously dismissed student. "I think what she was trying to say," but by then I was stuck in character. I cut her off with "Don't speak for others!" I misconstrued the ensuing laughter to mean universal recognition of my inept acting. It was only when Missy suddenly bolted out the door that I was jolted into the awareness of how unsafe the classroom had become.

Horrified, I stopped dead in my tracks then nodded approval at Sue who motioned that she was going to check on Missy. She exited. Not knowing what to do I blurted, "I was just acting. You knew that right?" I saw lots of nods, some knowing smiles, but just as many expressions of uncertainty. I gesture for a timeout in football fashion and sit down. I take a deep breath. "How you guys doing?" More nods. "I scared you didn't I?" More nods. "Do you think Missy is okay?" I ask, not wanting to abandon the rest of the class. More nods, but even more shoulder shrugs. "I hope she'll come back," I say "but I trust that she will do what she needs to do." I was talking more to myself than to the students. Truth was, I did not have a clue what to say or do.

After what seemed a very long silence, the wisdom of one of my beloved teachers came to me. Whenever encountered with a tough situation—find a way to talk about it. I invited the students to express their feelings. Some asserted that they knew right away what was going on and found it amusing.

Some vacillated back and forth between amusement and anxiety, others were bewildered. Some were worried for me and wanted to help but didn't know how. A few were really angry that I would do such a thing. It took all my energy to just hear them out and not try to defend my actions.

Missy and Sue returned. The tracks of her tears were readily apparent, Missy said she was okay but needed to leave. While she and Sue pack up her books, I asked her to come and see me later. She agreed readily, then left. Sue sat down and says Missy is upset because she has always been sensitive about talking more than others in the class. Baffled, I did a quick internal check—does she talk more than anyone else? That is not my assessment, but now I grasp why she looked so wounded. My arrow struck her Achilles' tendon.

The rest of the class and I talked for a while longer. I confessed that I was the instigator of the infectious emotion that overwhelmed us, and took responsibility for having violated what should have been a safe place. Noting my remorse, some students immediately melt with forgiveness, others are nonchalant; others still looked annoyed or otherwise upset with me. With about 20 minutes of class time remaining it's apparent we'd said as much as we could and I excused the students.

I dashed down to one trusted colleague's office and confessed my sin. The students who had just left my class were scheduled to reconvene in her research course in just 15 minutes. I wanted to prepare her for any residual fallout, but in the security of her presence, I melted down. She assured me that I am not the worst teacher ever, and ponders the likelihood of the students' attending to what she has planned. She decides to begin her class by acknowledging the turmoil in my class and gives the students the option of not meeting. They readily take her up on the offer—no surprise.

The experience really humbled me; in the immediate aftermath, it was for the worse possibly, but overall, it was for the better. I was a bit inhibited for the rest of the semester and engaged in fewer role-playing antics than I normally would have. Missy did come to talk with me individually and shared her concern that her classmates perceived her as a monopolizer. I doubt that my assurance that I did not regard her as such made any difference, but there was no change in her level of class participation. When the issue of safety came up in the context of subsequent course topics, I sometimes referred back to the contagiousness of emotion we had experienced earlier without again precipitating chaos.

The comedienne Carol Burnett is credited with saying that comedy is just tragedy plus time. Time has helped me to see how comical the situation was, especially the part where I allowed my distress to get the students out of their research class. Most of the students were not that affected by the experience. Being able to laugh at myself has helped me to see where I went astray. I had prior knowledge that four of the students in the class had been diagnosed with anxiety disorders (Missy and Sue among them), and I had tried this theatrical stunt far earlier than in previous semesters. The students had not yet trusted me enough for me to pull such a punch.

Colleen always says you can learn just as much from a bad role model as a good one. I'd rather be a good role model, and I hope that most of the time I am. Nonetheless, I am grateful for the humility that comes with acknowledging that knowledge and experience do not provide immunity from making mistakes.

Each of the story forms described so far allows our students some access into what it means to live a life with chronic illness. The grand narratives, deriving principally from the required texts and other assigned readings, are basically flat. The subsequent kinds of stories open students to fuller dimensions and greater depths of providing whole person care. In the artificiality of the classroom, they help evoke the thinking, feeling, and even behavioral responses students will need when faced with *real* clients in the *real* world. Including guest presenters in our course schema gives students a chance to interact with those who either have personal experience with chronic illness or provide care to those who do. It allows us an opportunity to express the college value of partnership, and it allows the students to ask questions they are afraid to raise with clients or with their professors.

STORIES IN THE FLESH

As with role-playing and other theatrical devices, relying on guests involves some risk. Like the old television commercial touting the cathartic benefits of prunes, we continually ask "Is one enough, are four too many?" Colleen sometimes fantasizes about composing the medical-surgical component entirely of guest speakers, each presenting their experience in living with _____ (fill in the blank). We have no shortage of available, relevant, and fascinating speakers, and no specific formula for determining the right number or mix. Student evaluations over the years have, however, led us to conclude that course continuity and student interest tends to break down if either one of us has more than three guests a semester in our individual components.

We have heard from enough experts or folks with amazing stories whose unfamiliarity with our course objectives or with public speaking made for boring, irrelevant, or confusing presentations to be cautious about turning our classroom over to just anybody. Luckily, we can be very selective and now have a slate of reliable, engaging personalities who are ongoing partners in our teaching endeavors. In any given semester, we tend to bring in new presenters for no more than a class period or two. Although each presenter has a particular content area that they address, due to student interactions and questions, repeat performances are never the same.

The stories of our visiting colleagues magnify what we can show students about whole person care through the lenses of caregiver concerns, self-regulation, and stigma. For example, two fellow teachers at the college who have undergone organ transplantation share very different tales of the ups and downs with their health and their health care providers. Their gratitude for the lives they would not be living without modern technology helps illustrate the benefits of the biomedical model. Their strict medication regimens and associated side-effects suggest the down-side and stimulates discussion of the nurse's role in helping clients do cost-benefit analyses in discerning treatment options. That both have the personal fortitude and essential financial and interpersonal resources to allow successful transplantation calls into question the equity of who does or does not qualify for second chances in life.

Whether by design or fate, the greatest majority of our guests are nurses. Some of them deal with chronic illness as part of their work and/or have personal experience with it. An advance practice nurse hired by a local hospital to design and implement a discharge program for people with congestive heart failure spoke about strategies he developed to prevent the frequent recurrent hospitalizations often experienced by this population. Hearing how the program has improved client outcomes and saved the institution thousands of dollars helps students understand the meaning of tertiary care and the power nurses have to enhance the lives of those living with chronic illness.

Another individual, whose nursing career was cut short by incapacitating depression, came to our class in her current role as the coordinator for a mental health consumer advocacy program. Her upbeat presentation belied the students' misconceptions that people with mental illness never get better. Also defying stereotypical views, a high powered nurse manager responsible for a local multiservice mental-health program educated the class about anxiety and dissociative disorders by sharing how his somewhat turbulent adolescence landed him in Viet Nam at age 19. After hearing his story of being taken hostage by a psychotic fellow-American soldier during his first week there, students had a visceral sense of how trauma figures in the development of post traumatic stress disorder (PTSD).

Each semester some of the guest speakers know the students and vice versa. A member of our nursing faculty shared her family's rocky journey through the mental-health system trying to get services for her brother, who was diagnosed with schizophrenia. Colleen became a guest lecturer in Pamela's class, Nursing Care of the Client With a Mental Disorder of Childhood or Adolescence. She talked about the challenges her son Adam and the whole family face as a result of his severe attention deficit and hyperactivity disorder. This willingness to be vulnerable in front of one's students promotes a sense of connection, underscores the pervasiveness of chronic illness, and models how candid discussion of the joys and burdens of tending to a loved one with a stigmatized condition can reduce caregiver strain.

Such vulnerability and its concomitant benefits are also apparent when the visiting scholar comes from the ranks of the learners. Three of our presenters are previous students who come back to share knowledge and expertise gained in the courses and from powerful personal experience. Carrie readies students for the chronic illness courses by helping Pamela teach a section on crisis intervention in NRS 310. Her extensive understanding of suicide prevention and intervention came as the result of her only sibling taking his own life at age 21. Her presentation made clear both the devastation that follows such loss and how bringing meaning to that occurrence promotes healing. It also made students acutely aware of their own susceptibility to stress and of the importance of taking care of themselves as they learn how to care for others.

Similarly, Greg's frank discussion of his long history of substance abuse and how it has several times threatened his professional license, awakened students to potential pitfalls in nursing. Posting a "résumé" of the 20-some drugs he has abused along with the amounts taken at the height of his drug career on the chalkboard and discussing how readily he could access and use them on the job conveyed volumes about the issue of impaired providers. It also drove home the point that the incidence of substance abuse is greater among nurses than it is in the general population.

Maradee taught about end-of-life concerns with a PowerPoint presentation filled with photos she took in an Edgewood art course and memories of being a hospice volunteer. Her conversion from what she describes as an arrogant do-gooder to a humble servant conveyed a message more readily heard from a peer than a professor.

The stories of these three students-turned-teachers appear in greater depth in chapter 6. What they have to say to their successors is especially powerful, because (1) they can empathize with the current lot of the students, (2) their accomplishments are so inspiring, and (3) they are incredibly articulate in expressing how they have been transformed by their experiences. Their successes convince the incumbent students that they too can survive the chronic illness courses, and stokes their desire to contribute to society in equally significant ways.

That all of the above mentioned teaching partners speak firsthand of the despair of losing one's self-regulatory capacity, the effects of living with a stigmatized condition, and/or the stresses inherent in nursing gives them great credibility in students' eyes. Although it is not uncommon for the students to ask after a guest's departure, "What do we really need to know for the test?" their course evaluations indicate that the stories shared by these amazing people have transformative effects. In all likelihood, many students would say our most regular coconspirers, John and Adrian, who were introduced in chapter 2, have the most profound effect on them, though. They are indeed some of our most provocative coteachers, in the most positive way.

Since the inception of the theory course, John and Adrian have shared what it means to live a life under the shadow of HIV+ status. Both men have met the diagnostic criteria for AIDS at some point in their illness, and as is apparent in chapter 2, both manage their illness, and lives, quite differently. They candidly discuss their lifestyle and the abuses it has often earned them, even in the health care field where they were both employed for many years. Students listen attentively throughout their discourse, unable to comprehend how stereotypically negative views of homosexuality could ever apply to such wise and entertaining sages. They wonder as well why two people who openly acknowledge the physical toll it takes on them persist in coming to NRS 340 twice a year. They require a minimum of 14 hours of sleep a night to function and it takes them a day or two to regain their stamina after a 2-hour speaking gig in our class.

The generosity of our visiting scholars is unmistakable, especially in light of the fact that they receive no monetary remuneration. Each one is uniquely qualified and suited to teach about some aspect of chronic illness and whole person care, and each one shares the commonality of being altruistically motivated to do so. Thus, it is not so surprising when our expressions of gratitude are met with their thanks for providing a forum that allows them to help shape future nursing practice. The importance of this is particularly evident in John and Adrian's summation of why they come to speak to us.

John

So why do Adrian and I agree to speak out? What do we have to offer that is so special? I don't know that we have anything unique beyond ourselves to offer. There are as many other unique stories that can be told. We have grown together and reached significant points of commonality in our process that has placed us in the unique position of being available to speak out; it is a matter of circumstances, chance, and choice.

I think it is important to realize when you are dealing with an individual with an illness that they are so much more than their illness. Individuals carry their past and present on their shoulders.

I ask you to beware of judging others. There are behaviors that are clearly unacceptable and these limits need to be set for all individuals, but these limits will seldom be the issue you need to deal with. More likely, you will be confronted with some individual who stimulates a gut response from you. In our case, you may share the gut response that gay people are sinners and choose their identity, rather than being born that way.

You may have a deepseated belief that we are "unclean" or are "untouchables" and undeserving of care and concern. You may have grown up around these attitudes, believe yourself to be immune to them, and still find they have affected your interaction with the individual in question. Something about the way someone is dressed or cares for themselves may influence you to judge them in a particular manner. It's not that we don't all do those automatically, but if you are unaware of it and act out of this blindness, you are not caring for an individual. Instead, you are caring for a preconception—*your* preconception.

Live my life better than I did, and then you may have the right to criticize or judge me.

Adrian

I speak to educate. Education is a key part to understanding. Bigotry and hatred are usually the products of ignorance, and by speaking to nursing classes I hope to make vague concepts a reality.

I remember my first days in nursing, I was afraid of just about everything and every patient around me. One thing I have learned through my personal experience with a chronic disease is that there isn't a thing that you can ask or say to me that hasn't run through my head. I think about death, I think about being sick and disabled. I sometimes think about being hooked up to machines keeping me alive and wonder what kind of life that would be for me and for the people that love me. I get angry when a medical professional announces that they know what I'm going through. That's impossible, how can any of you know what it is like for me to live through this?

None of you know the devastating affects the AIDS pandemic has had on my life. I'm not sure, but I wonder how many of you have lost hundreds of friends, watched countless young people die from a disease that your government and president wouldn't even name? Do you understand the depth of my anger and hurt? Do you understand the shame and guilt that religious groups can cast upon you for loving who you love or being who you are? It runs deep. Do you understand that after listening to medical professionals joke about their patient's sexual orientation there is a certain basic mistrust that I carry with me just as surely as I carry my pj's and toothbrush?

Twice a year, I come in and discuss things with you that most people try to keep private. Why? There are an infinite number of answers to this question, but I have only a few reasons to make myself this vulnerable. I come in and lay my soul bare so that you can safely ask questions that are knocking about your brain. I come in because right now, there is an alarming trend among people to put AIDS/HIV on the back burner because there are drugs. AIDS/HIV still kills. AIDS/HIV still makes life incredibly difficult and still makes one sick as hell.

There is no cure. I hear how excited people are about a possible vaccine. I'm not very excited; a vaccine won't do a thing for me or the millions of people like me that have AIDS/HIV. I speak to you because no matter how much information there is about odds and chances of getting AIDS/HIV, in reality, when you get it, the odds and chances are meaningless. I speak to you because if I had a genetic disease I might seem more acceptable to you. I speak to you because someday, you could be taking care of me, and hopefully you will remember me and give me that extra care that may just get me over the hump.

I speak to you because I know your instructor would hunt me down if I didn't. Besides, I get taken to lunch if I do a good job; at the very least I get coffee and snacks.

I speak to you because after almost 20 years, AIDS/HIV has taken its toll on me, and I don't have the energy to do the big-ticket items. I speak to you because I can. I also speak for selfish reasons. Speaking makes me feel like I am doing something in the war on AIDS/HIV. It makes me feel good. I speak for my own well-being. If I do good things, good things will happen to me, I think it is called karma. I tell you my stories so that you can put a face on this most evil disease.

CONCLUSION

The stories we share in the theory course are important for at least two primary reasons. First, they allow us to weave textbook information into meaningful contexts; that is, the experiences of whole people leading real lives both encumbered and enhanced by chronic illness. Stories address tertiary prevention, daily management, family concerns, and nursing roles in a way that students can readily grasp. The tales of trial, tribulation, and even triumph we share will move some of our graduates to work in the chronic care arena. A greater number may well opt for acute care settings, but the numerous personal accounts in the chronic illness theory course of how nurses can make or break a life after discharge will hopefully remind them of the importance of listening carefully to the patient's story.

The second reason case stories are important is because students remember Joe, Uncle Lee, John Nash, Carrie, Maradee, Greg, Adrian, and John, and the cast of other characters they meet in the course. They will have to review the content presented on any given topic area in order to pass the NCLEX exam, but they do not forget the stories of disease progression, its long-term consequences and impact on family, and the associated losses. Students remember the narrative long after they have forgotten the minute details of the nursing management of any disease entity.

Charmez (1991) describes the experience of chronic illness as encompassing good days and bad days. "A good day means minimal intrusiveness of illness, maximal control over mind, body, and actions and greater choice of activities. . . . Illness remains in the background, whereas a bad day means the opposite. Illness and regimen take center stage. On a bad day, people cannot ignore or easily minimize illness" (p. 50).

Similarly, our teaching consists of good days and bad days. On bad days we get stuck in singular thinking and the myth that covering the content means we must actually vocalize every relevant concept and concern related to the topic at hand in order for our students to understand. A good day is when the stories we share allow the content and process of our teaching to fit together seamlessly.

REFERENCES

Albom, M. (1997). *Tuesdays with Morrie.* New York: Doubleday.

Beam, A. (2003). *Gracefully insane.* Cambridge, MA: Perseus Books.

Charmez, K. (1991). *Good days, bad days.* New Brunswick, NJ: Rutgers University Press.

Chinn, P. L., & Kramer, M. K. (1999). *Theory and nursing: Integrated knowledge and development.* St. Louis: Mosby.

Clandinin, D. J., & Connelly, F. M. (1994). Personal experience methods. In N. K. Denzin & Y. S. Lincoln (Eds.), *Handbook of qualitative research* (pp. 413–427). Thousand Oaks, CA: Sage Publications.

Deegan, P. (1993). Recovering our sense of value after being labeled. *Journal of Psychosocial Nursing, 31*(4), 7–11.

Ellsworth, E. (1997). *Teaching positions.* New York: Teachers College Press.

Farrell, S. P., Harmon, R. B., & Hastings, S. (1998). Nursing management of acute psychotic episodes. *Nursing Clinics of America, 33*(1), 187–199.

Gere, A. G., Ruggles, C. F., Howes, A., Roop, L., & Schaafsma, D. (1992). *Language and reflection: An integrated approach to teaching English.* New York: Macmillian Publishing.

Miller, M. E., & Dzurec, L. C. (1993). The power of the name. *Advances in Nursing Science, 15*(3), 15–22.

Munhall, P. L. (1993). 'Unknowing': Toward another pattern of knowing in nursing. *Nursing Outlook, 41,* 125–128.

Nagai-Jacobson, M. G., & Burkhardt, M. A. (1996). Viewing persons as stories: A perspective for holistic care. *Alternative Therapies, (2)*4, 54–58.

Palmer, P. (1990). *The active life.* San Francisco: Harper and Row.

Paul, R., & Willsen, J. (1993). *Critical thinking: From an ideal evolves an imperative.* Santa Rosa, CA: The Foundation for Critical Thinking.

Silva, M. C., Sorrell, J. M., & Sorrell, C. D. (1995). From Carper's patterns of knowing to ways of being: An ontological philosophical shift in nursing. *Advances in Nursing Science, 18*(1), 1–13.

Van Manen, M. (1990). *Researching lived experience: Human science for action sensitive pedagogy.* Albany, NY: State University of New York Press.

Vella, J. (2002). *Learning to listen, learning to teach.* San Francisco: Jossey.

5

Teaching the Clinical Component

Nursing has its roots in holistic humus, and it is currently popular for a variety of health care disciplines to espouse the importance of addressing the whole person. Nonetheless, care continues to be dominated by the medical model and the emphasizing of acute intervention that is, most often, hospital-based. Caring for people with chronic illness fosters an appreciation for the fact that health can exist even in the face of illness and that promoting the former and diminishing the later requires a comprehensive continuum of care.

Upon successful completion of Edgewood's nursing program, many of our students will find themselves in acute care settings, at least initially. Understanding what it means to live a life with chronic illness and how to provide whole person care are essential even though our students will return to the hospital in the subsequent semester and may well work there after graduation. Thoughtful decision-making and discharge planning in acute care hinges on recognition that for the patient, life extends well beyond the confines of today's restricted hospital stays.

The intent of our chronic illness clinical course (NRS 341) is to provide extensive and varied opportunities to apply, with support and supervision, the knowledge conveyed in its theory companion course. In other words, clinical students get to practice what we preach in the theory course. This chapter discusses some of the challenges and rewards of teaching clinical practice focused on helping people with chronic illness live the lives *they* want. First, we identify the course objectives. An overview of the course design, including its structure, clinical site selection, and faculty considerations follow. The details of teaching whole-person care for those experiencing chronic challenges to their physical and/or mental health come later in the chapter, along with discussion of the specific learning activities we employ. The chapter concludes with discussion of student assessment.

COURSE OBJECTIVES

In the theory course we share stories of self-regulation, stigma, and caregiver concerns as they relate to chronic illness. In the clinical course we live them. Like the theory course, the clinical course was designed to meet specific objectives that derive from and are intertwined with the six curricular strands of caring, health, client/person, professional nursing, environment, and critical thinking.

As was noted in chapter 4, the course objectives serve as a kind of compass marking the place of each course in the undergraduate curriculum and guiding decisions about the type and nature of the learning experiences students will engage in. The clinical course has six objectives:

1. Apply nursing process to maximize client functioning.
2. Advocate for needed resources to assure continuity of care.
3. Collaborate with multidisciplinary teams to promote client participation in treatment.
4. Demonstrate commitment and accountability for clinical decision making.
5. Develop self as therapeutic agent while maintaining respect for client individuality.
6. Make clinical decisions that reflect consideration of context.

The essence of the clinical course is *practice, practice,* and *practice.* This is a clinical course in which practicing the skills necessary to help clients create their own stories of living well with illness is tantamount. Some of the skills are technical ones, like starting IVs or administering medications, but the greater emphasis is on organizational and interpersonal abilities. Students practice over and over again the skills of attending to the whole person, regardless of the presenting problem or the arena in which it arises, and of coordinating and providing care for psychosocial-spiritual concerns as well as bodily needs.

When applied to patients, clients, members, consumers, residents, and neighbors (just some of the terms used to describe the people we work with in clinical) the lenses of self-regulation, caregiver concerns, and stigma converge at a new focal point, thus opening students to the possibility that living a life with chronic illness can be one characterized by wellness. This notion of wellness draws on a conception of health and illness as existing on two separate but overlapping continua that allow individuals to have varying degrees of each concurrently (Greenberg, 1995). Magnification of these continua reveals a series of circular *health dots*, each of which is comprised of physical, mental, social and spiritual facets. Integration of the facets at any level of health or illness into a coherent whole is called wellness. While wellness is always a positive state and illness is always negative, they can coexist. Wellness is characterized as vitality or zest for life (Greenberg, 1995).

Being able to recognize wellness is not a skill that comes readily to students after a semester of providing nursing care for acutely ill patients, let alone a lifetime of thinking that health and illness are mutually exclusive phenomena. The clinical course requires students to shift from a pathogenic orientation to a salutogenic one. This later paradigm recognizes that while we will all ultimately die, a degree of health exists as long as there is life. A pathogenic orientation asks what causes disease, while a salutogenic one questions what moves people toward health ease (Antonovsky, 1987), or wellness. The latter attitude legitimizes students asking questions like "What are this person's strengths?" and "What evidence of wellness is apparent?" in addition to, or sometimes even in the place of, a staid barrage of illness oriented inquiries.

In the clinical course students become acutely aware of the "language of deficit" mentioned in chapter 3. This frees them to think more in terms of client assets and to practice the skills of engaging clients in care planning and doing cost-benefit analyses of treatment options. Students come to the course somewhat proficient in nursing process but have been preoccupied with identifying problems and the appropriate nursing interventions to remedy them. And, they have become accustomed to thinking about nursing interventions as something to do to or for a patient. As educators, we are sometimes guilty of perpetuating this thinking when students approach us in a clinical setting with an identified problem and our first response is, *"What are you going to do?"* Although appropriate in some settings, this may undermine care when dealing with individuals with chronic illness.

"What are you going to do?" is best suited for situations requiring immediate attention. Helping students differentiate between imminent need and concerns more responsive to a "tincture of time" is part of teaching chronic illness management. Often, the most relevant response lies in *being with* the client rather than doing to or for. Being with involves listening to the client's concerns, acknowledging his or her situation, and being mindful that there may not be an immediate solution or any solution at all. Being with is a skill difficult for students to

comprehend and for many nurses to master. There are no tasks to do, no pieces of equipment to monitor or hide behind. The nurse is the intervention. Perhaps the most difficult and highest level skill students practice in this class is that of therapeutic presence.

COURSE DESIGN

Helping students to meet the above-described objectives is challenging. NRS 341 is structured to give them the chance to work *with* individuals and families encountering complex long-term health problems, to engage in multidisciplinary collaboration, and experience firsthand what it means to provide continuity of care.

Like the theory course, the clinical course is composed of two interdependent components. Academia frequently separates nursing knowledge into compartments, such as medical-surgical and psychiatric-mental health nursing. While these are convenient for descriptive purposes and facilitate learning to some degree, they tend to obscure what Palmer (1998) calls the "hidden wholeness." We continually struggle with how to organize NRS 341 so as to optimize student mastery of a variety of technical, practical, and interpersonal skills and still do justice to whole-person care. The resolution to this dilemma lies in continually reminding ourselves of the theoretical frame delineated in chapter 3.

Structure

The clinical course is four-credit course that engages students in 12 hours of weekly clinical practice for 16 weeks. Eight hours weekly are devoted to caring for individuals facing chronic physical illness who are on a rehabilitation or sub-acute unit in a hospital or long-term care facility, or in a hospice setting. The balance of the 12 hours is divided up over the course of the semester to provide students with a variety of institution and community-based experiences emphasizing care of individuals with chronic mental illness.

We refer to the two components of the course as the medical-surgical component and the psychosocial-spiritual component. Each of these is described in more detail later. Colleen has primary responsibility for the first component, and Pamela for the latter. We are aware that these designations may unfortunately imply a distinction between physical and mental health concerns replicating the mind/body dualism we seek to overcome. In spite of the limits of our language, we hold to the belief that *"there is much 'physical' in 'mental' disorders and much 'mental' in 'physical'disorders"* (American Psychiatric Association, 1994, p. XXI).

While problems in the physical facet of health tend to be the catalyst for care in the settings where the medical-surgical component takes place, and concerns about the mental facet are most often the reason for developing therapeutic relationships in the psychosocial-spiritual component of the course, both provide ample opportunity to practice whole-person care. All the assumptions described in chapter 3 hold equally in both parts of the course, as do the following additional ones. We assert that psychiatric disorder increases vulnerability to physical illness and vice versa. Similarly, psychosocial and spiritual effects clearly accompany physical illness, and their behavioral or psychological manifestations can complicate, help resolve, or enhance coping with it.

The maximum course enrollment is 35. During the registration process, students are placed in clinical sections of no more than seven each, according to their first or second choices. Thus, in any given semester there may be as many as five clinical sections. Each section has one instructor for the medical-surgical component and another for the psychosocial-spiritual component. They functional fairly autonomously, although there are times in the semester when learning activities relevant to the psychosocial-spiritual component bring together small groups of students from different clinical sections or gather the entire group. Instructor collaboration is essential to smooth course functioning and thus quarterly faculty meetings are held to address curricular and student issues.

Site Selection

Location! Location! Location! Why is location such an important factor, not only in selecting real estate, but also in choosing an appropriate clinical site? What is it about a particular location that makes it potentially better than another? How are clinical sites chosen and for what reasons? These are all very important questions and deserve considerable deliberation.

Selection of a clinical site is a multivariate process involving more complex issues than the mere composition of the clinical population. Consideration must also be given to faculty competence, willingness of staff to work with students, availability of the clinical site as well as travel time, reputation of the facility, and client census. We are fortunate that our geographical area is rich enough in resources to allow the course objectives to drive our site selection. What we look for are environments, physical and social, in which our students have the opportunity to participate in stories of whole person care.

Some faculty might argue that acute care settings offer ample opportunity for students to care for clients with chronic illness. We agree, to a degree. Clearly, hospitals are filled with people experiencing diabetic complications, heart failure, respiratory problems, or mental health crises. We argue, however, that while such locations provide exposure to chronic illness management, the focus on medical management of exacerbations of chronic illness makes it more difficult to see the larger picture. It is not that we dispute that acute care experiences are vital and necessary to undergraduate nursing education. We just see them as rightly constituting only one piece of the entire clinical pie.

All too often, sociopolitical forces create a "treat 'em and street 'em" mentality in acute care that obscures for students the importance of thinking holistically. Experienced nurses may grasp that notion, but it is difficult for junior-level nursing students to see goals beyond resolution of the medical or psychiatric problem that forced hospital admission when their contact with a given patient is limited to 8 hours. In the best scenario, they simply miss that long-standing problems likely precipitated admission and/or misconstrue that being more physically or mentally stable upon discharge to mean that the patient is "all better." More concerning is the potential for students to resent how "frequent flyers" or "chronics" bog down the health care system. If this is the only exposure students have to people living with chronic illness, they are prone to develop a frighteningly short-sighted, extremely contagious, and difficult to eradicate mindset that the patient is to blame for the system's woes. Here are a few examples: An individual receiving chronic dialysis comes to the center 20 pounds over her normal weight—blame the patient for not doing a better job with her food and fluid restrictions; a person with chronic lung disease is admitted with pneumonia—blame the patient for not getting his pneumonia shot; a WWII veteran is admitted for detoxification after a week long drinking binge—blame the patient for having such poor self control.

More astute students realize the futility of blaming patients for scenarios like those just noted. They recognize that the quick fix premise in acute care precludes having sufficient time to address or resolve larger patient concerns. They are at risk for the disillusionment and disempowerment that comes with concluding that chronic illness management is a *revolving-door* phenomenon. One reason this posture can readily develop is that acute care does not provide sufficient opportunity to understand the complexities of living a life with chronic illness. Given its highly structured, strictly controlled environment, acute care is akin to an experimental design, where nothing is left to chance. For most individuals, living a life with a chronic illness is more parallel to interpretive study. Students need time to get to know the people they are caring for before they can appreciate the multidimensional challenges they face.

Where, then, might students have a better experience of caring for individuals living with chronic illness? We have not yet found a single place that encompasses all the key characteristics we look for, so we make use of a variety of clinical sites, both institution and community-based.

We want our students to work with people facing physical, psychosocial, and spiritual challenges to their health and to have an opportunity to develop longer-term relationships with them. This latter requirement is the most central to the clinical course, and it applies to both the medical-surgical and psychosocial-spiritual components.

When nursing students are assigned a new client each week, they do not get to see how issues are resolved and seldom feel the sense of mastery that comes with being involved in a client's care over time. A longer-term relationship allows the partnership necessary for whole-person care to evolve between client and student. As a partner, the student witnesses firsthand the barriers and challenges many clients face. This enhances their sensitivity to the complexity of living a life with chronic illness and makes them less condemnatory when individuals make different choices than they would. In the medical-surgical component of the course students take care of a patient for several weeks at a time, and in the psychosocial-spiritual component they interact with the same clients throughout an entire semester. One student's experience of being able to follow a patient after discharge from a rehabilitation unit where she was recuperating after a fall illustrates the profound impact such relationships can have on learning and care.

Irene and Katie

Irene was in her late 70s, and it took a team of social workers, nurses, home health aides, and a number of other helpers to stave off placement in a nursing home. She was adamant about returning to her apartment in the low-income neighborhood that was home to an odd mix of vulnerable seniors and younger people with physical and mental disabilities. Her mild dementia and severe anxiety kept her from leaving her apartment except on rare occasions. Though she could ambulate with a walker, she much preferred her wheelchair, and she liked to be pushed. She resisted all suggestions that she dine at the senior meal program just adjacent to her building, preferring to depend on Meals-On-Wheels for nourishment. A severe hiatal hernia caused her much discomfort and regular bouts of abstinence from eating. She wasn't reliable about taking her medication and was vehemently opposed to any surgical intervention. Particularly bad dentition and a total terror of dentists exacerbated the problem. Coupled with an inability to manage her diabetes independently, her very bossy manner had earned her the distinction of a *dual diagnosis—manipulative and noncompliant.*

Irene's case manager was opposed to having a nursing student named Katie come to visit her most problematic client. She regarded Katie as just one more sap Irene could play off against other well-intentioned do-gooders. She relented, though, when there was no one else available to accompany Irene to a long-scheduled dentist's appointment. The case manager wanted to capitalize on the fact that Irene, to everyone's amazement, had agreed to go.

Miraculously, Irene was immediately smitten with Katie's youthful cheeriness and the fact that they shared a passion for butterflies. This seemed to make the case manager even more doubtful of Katie's abilities, but they worked cooperatively to make the necessary travel arrangements and prepare Irene for the excursion.

The day of the appointment Katie allowed plenty of time, but, despite her patient assistance, Irene was so nervous that it took even longer than usual for her to get ready. The weather wasn't cooperating either. It had been sleeting for several hours, and even with a frighteningly speedy cab ride through icy streets they were almost 20 minutes late for the appointment. Adding insult to injury, a terse receptionist greeted them with a derogatory comment about tardiness and pushed a clipboard full of paperwork into Katie's hands.

The receptionist tried to turn them away when Katie didn't have the necessary insurance verification. Fearful that she'd never get Irene to return, Katie insisted that the receptionist call the case manager. By a stroke of luck, she was in, and emboldened by Katie's assertiveness, insisted on speaking directly to the dentist. By now Irene quivered uncontrollably, but the case manger's pleas and Katie's assurance that if the dentist would just let her hold Irene's hand she'd be all right, forced him to agree to proceed with the examination. Katie tried several times to get the dentist to speak directly to Irene but gave up as he persisted in talking to her as if she were a parent and Irene her incompetent child.

The next day in NRS 340 Katie commented, "If they only knew what we went through to get to that appointment, I think they would have been a little nicer to Irene." She and several of her peers vowed that they would not allow any of their future clients to suffer the kind of degradation Irene had that day. The ordeal seemed to solidify the bond between Irene and Katie and earned Katie the case manager's esteem.

To celebrate Irene's courage and help her overcome the winter blahs, Katie arranged an outing to a local botanical garden that had a glassed-in pavilion filled with live butterflies. Everyone was surprised when Irene agreed to go and delighted that the planned day, though very cold, was filled with sunshine. Katie and Irene spent 4 hours just sitting together surrounded by butterflies and soaking up the rays. They had a passerby take some photos of them, which Katie gave Irene as a goodbye gift at the end of the semester.

At the beginning of the next semester we heard that Irene's health had rapidly deteriorated over the winter. She died alone in her apartment, apparently as the result of a stroke. On her nightstand the case manager found a picture of Katie and Irene laughing and looking with amazement at a large brightly colored butterfly perched in Irene's hand. The case manager was so struck by the contrast to Irene's usually dour expression that she was moved at the funeral to tuck the memento into her casket.

When we told Katie about Irene's death she said, "I know some people had a hard time with Irene, but I really liked being with her. I think she was just trying to live her life the way she wanted."

Beyond allowing for longer-term relationships, Irene and Katie's story exemplifies several other crucial characteristics we look for in clinical sites. Because we want these relationships to be therapeutic, that is, to promote the wellness of those being served, the sites need to present opportunities for meaningful interaction around real concerns. Real concerns can be physical, mental, social, or spiritual needs that are not being met by the client himself or herself, or by other caregivers. Meaningful interaction implies relationships that are mutually beneficial for the direct recipient of care and/or other caregivers trying to help meet the recipient's needs and the student. We intentionally seek out underserved and/or particular challenging populations to maximize the potential for contributing to the wellness of those who might otherwise not receive care. We go where our students will be allowed to actually practice, practice, practice—not just observe—concrete and more abstract nursing skills.

Whole-person care entails being open to all aspects of an individual's life and collaborating on matters beyond the limited scope of illness management. Katie was involved in the continuum of care Irene required, from an inpatient experience all the way to organizing transportation and just hanging out with her. As Irene's advocate, she not only had a hand in moving her toward wellness, but got to practice teamwork with other caregivers who were somewhat resistant, thereby enhancing her own confidence. She also got an invaluable lesson about how stigma and economics can impinge on treatment. These are the kinds of opportunities we expect our clinical sites to offer.

Coming from acute care to chronic illness, students are most accustomed to nurses performing activities mandated by medical orders. They understand treatment to entail tangible procedures or to follow written protocols. They have not yet come to fully understand that nursing process is not linear, or that, as nurses, their work will not be limited to problem identification and delivery of discrete corporal nursing interventions. Clinical experiences in NRS 341 are intended to help them grasp that what on the surface appears to be a social outing is really an opportunity to assess receptive and expressive language function, problem-solving and functional abilities, personal hygiene, mood states, and much more. Similarly, having lunch at a meal site provides a wealth of information regarding physical stamina, swallow ability, cognitive processing, appetite, and food preferences. Initially such activities have students questioning their role as nurses, but when given a chance to collaborate with a multidisciplinary team, they come to appreciate a broader scope of nursing practice, one that encompasses all the components of caring for an individual and his/her family—a scope of practice based on the concept of whole-person care.

The presence of positive nurse role models—both those in more and in less traditional roles—is also a factor we consider in site selection. Although there is an Edgewood nursing faculty member on site with the students for the majority of their clinical time, they are often in the company of staff. Chapter 4 noted Colleen's wisdom that one can learn from a bad examples as well as a good ones, but we find that students learn more readily and happily where they are welcome and when they get to witness directly what quality care looks like. We have found as well that when we bring our students to help out in significant ways, staff members are far more receptive. The clinical sites we use all share the characteristic of allowing students to function as full and equal members in the care team.

We have found that clinical staff attitudes toward and approaches to students are often mirrored in their relationships with their clientele. We seek learning environments in which our students can actualize the college's commitment to service, partnership, truth, justice, and compassion. At the most basic level, that means choosing clinical sites where positive regard for the people being served is obvious in the care culture.

Faculty Considerations

Like all accredited baccalaureate nursing programs, ours requires faculty to have educational preparation at least at the masters level in nursing, relevant clinical and teaching experience, active licensure, and current competency in the skills to be taught. We expect as well that those who teach with us have an understanding and appreciation for a liberal arts education and an investment in the mission of the college. They must also have some familiarity with the entire undergraduate-nursing curriculum. Further criteria we consider in choosing clinical faculty are implicit in the preceding discussion of site selection and in the curricular framework described in chapter 3. Anyone teaching in the clinical course has to buy into whole person care and its concomitant premises and be able to keep it at the forefront even in settings where the focus might be elsewhere. Whether teaching in the medical-surgical or psychosocial-spiritual component of the course, each instructor must keep all the dimensions of health in mind when overseeing student practice.

The way the course is structured, at periods when enrollment is maximized and we are operating five clinical sections with seven students each, we can have as many as seven faculty members involved in one semester. As course coordinators, we oversee the work of adjunct faculty as well as teach clinical sections of our own. There have been times when low enrollment has meant we were the only ones teaching the course. We look at those times somewhat nostalgically, because they allowed us to lavish more attention on our students and the people they were caring for. Collaborating was a breeze, because the two of us share a passion for whole-person care and a vision for making it happen. Communicating about student progress or clinical site concerns, and negotiating workload, was simplified as well when we were a teaching dyad.

With potentially five proportional positions and inevitable turnover, we devote a fair amount of time to orienting and mentoring new people, serving as links to the rest of the nursing faculty and the college at large, and mediating between students and part time instructors. The upside of having a full slate of colleagues is that students have exposure to a wider spectrum of ideas and teaching styles. With a faculty team and a continual influx of personnel comes the energy and stimulation to develop new and creative teaching strategies and activities. Our course coordination role requires, though, that whatever innovative endeavors get pursued are consistent with the course objectives and our wellness orientation. Given the nursing profession's holistic roots, it is somewhat ironic that the latter requirement can be quite difficult for some faculty. While we expect that care in some clinical sites will derive principally from the prevalent medical model, clinical instructors have to be able to see beyond pathology and a cure mentality in order to help students understand what it means to live a life with chronic illness.

As a rule, we do not place students in clinical sites where they are employed. Trying to learn what it means to be a nurse gets compromised in settings where the student works as a nursing assistant or in some other position. Learning is diminished when she or he has to continually differentiate between role expectations or balance the desires of her or his teacher and coworkers. Similarly, such situations impinge on the gift of perspective students ordinarily bring to clinical. Being outside the status quo decreases students' self-consciousness and enhances their latitude as learners, because it allows them to innocently question standard practice. Our inclination is to apply these same tenets to adjunct faculty, but periodic shortages of qualified educators mean we sometimes bend them.

We want our faculty to be free from the constraints of teaching in settings where they are on staff. While familiarity with a given clinic or unit can provide a leg up in some senses, we have found that more often than not, faculty who play dual roles have a harder time staying focused on the course objectives. Ideally the faculty member serves as a mediator between the insider (i.e., staff) and outsider (i.e., student) view, constantly reorienting the two to the whole-person care orientation of the class. Thus, the faculty member must bring objectivity and the experience and expertise that grant credibility within the system where the clinical takes place.

Students get an intimate view of their instructors as role models. Chapter 4 noted that we challenge our students to challenge us as teachers, so we have to have faculty who do not feel a need to be infallible. It is equally important that they allow students to be students—in other words, to sometimes make mistakes or fail. An aura of perfection undermines student confidence and willingness to embrace new experiences or to think on their own. Students seem to have the most positive experiences when their instructors have a sense of humor, evidenced by a capacity to laugh with their students and at their own inevitable foibles. In clinical we seek to promote student self-awareness toward the end that they will be less self-conscious in their dealings with clients. This is facilitated by having faculty who are process oriented so they do not get stuck just teaching content and can help the students reflect on their experiences.

PSYCHOSOCIAL-SPIRITUAL COMPONENT

The psychosocial-spiritual component of the clinical course involves one third of the total required clinical hours for the course, or the equivalent of 4 hours per week for 16 weeks. We say the equivalent of 4 hours a week because the first half of the semester is front-loaded with more hours to help students adjust to what initially seem to be strange environments, and to ready them to do more independent work later. Thus, minus time for holiday breaks, students spend a total of 60 hours of clinical time working with a specified population of individuals who have chronic mental illnesses, visiting and leading therapeutic groups, attending client-centered presentations and team meetings, and engaging in brief independent experiences that are tailored to their specific learning needs.

Milieu

Placements for the psychosocial-spiritual component of the course can vary from semester to semester, and from each other in terms of whether they are community or institutionally based. The key aims (Motives) and learning activities (Methods) described later, however, mandate what sort of physical sites are workable. Each small clinical group of seven students and one instructor has a primary post where they spend the greatest majority of time each semester. While students will be assigned to one or the other, they are required to participate in activities at both. There are several times during the semester when students from all clinical sections gather together to learn about forensic psychiatry, therapeutic groups, or the experience of having a mental illness, and to share what they have learned about the continuum of psychosocial-spiritual care.

At the present time, we are able to accommodate all of our students in two principal locations. The first is a subsidized housing project just down the street from the college. Students interact with residents from four different apartment complexes that share an on-site, 5-days-a-week meal program and a part-time health clinic. All of the residents live on fixed incomes. Thirty-seven percent of them are elderly, 66% have a mental disability, 52% have developmental disabilities, and 28% have significant drug or alcohol concerns. The residents live independently in their own apartments, although many receive supportive services from a variety of community agencies. The clinic nurse and a neighborhood-based parish nurse provide outreach to the residents, many of whom do not have reasonable access to basic health care services. These two nurses collaborate with the NRS 341 instructor to identify resident needs and ways to promote student learning by meeting them.

The second principal location is a medium security inpatient forensic psychiatric unit located at a nearby state hospital. The unit provides treatment for approximately 20 male patients who have a history of major mental illness and criminal activity. They are hospitalized involuntarily, and may remain from a few weeks to a number of years. Many of the patients also suffer from one or several chronic illnesses that are physical in nature. A multidisciplinary staff of nurses, psychiatrists, psychologists, social workers, and occupational and recreational therapists collaborate to provide a therapeutic milieu promoting patient rehabilitation and quality of life. The clinical instructor based there works with unit staff to assure that pursuit of the course objectives is a mutually beneficial process.

What these two seemingly disparate sites have in common is the population served within their confines. Both residents and patients face a plethora of physical, spiritual, social, and mental threats to wellness, but it is concerns in the latter two dimensions that evoke public interest in their health status. Some of the residents have spent time at the state hospital, though not necessarily in the forensic program. Some of the patients did live in or are now living in the housing project. Many of the other patients are mentally stable enough to be living independently in the community, but their crimes preclude this option.

Another similarity between the two sites we are currently using, and an essential requirement we have in considering any potential site for this aspect of NRS 341 is their ability to offer opportunities for the students to conduct wellness interviews and lead therapeutic groups. These two activities, described in more detail in the section titled Methods, are key in helping students achieve the specific aims of the psychosocial-spiritual component of the course, which are delineated under Motives.

In acute care, especially in general hospitals, clinicians reign supreme. The clinical sites for the psychosocial-spiritual component of the course place the students and their instructors on more foreign turf and require that they adapt their attitudes, expectations, and behaviors to those of multiple and diverse hosts. They undergo a shift in status from that of experts who tell patients what to do to that of informed practitioners who have something to offer only when they take the time to know the patients or residents and collaborate with them. They have to function without uniforms or other health care paraphernalia to hide behind. This becomes even more the case when, during the later half of the semester, students venture out on their own to visit a variety of mental health or hospice programs, therapeutic groups, and social service agencies.

Motives

In addition to the six course objectives, the psychosocial-spiritual component delineates five more circumscribed overlapping motives or aims. A sampling of student quotes from their written assignments and final self-evaluations helps illustrate how each of these is actualized.

Many students come to the chronic illness clinical course not only with stereotypical ideas about what it means to have a mental illness, but also about nursing in the mental-health field. One aim of this component of the course is to help students transcend stigmatized views of both. A second is to cultivate an appreciation for psychiatric nursing as both a clinical specialty *and* an integral aspect of all nursing. Though usually only a handful of students have interest in gaining the experience—and, in some cases, advanced education—necessary to practice the specialty of psychiatric nursing, all will need to function as psychiatric nurses in the second sense. That is to say, they will encounter mentally ill clients in every health care setting, and even mentally fit clients will have psychosocial and spiritual needs when their physical health is threatened—thus, they will need to be able to apply psychological theory to their practice regardless of the settings in which they find themselves. A recurring theme in student evaluations of the psychosocial-spiritual component of the course is that many students were skeptical of its value upon entering, but all steadfastly believed at the end of the semester that the experience would prove to be pivotal in their ability to provide whole person care no matter what type of nursing they will pursue.

The immense and ever-growing body of knowledge and skills that the baccalaureate student nurse (BSN) must master in order to graduate as a competent and safe generalist practitioner precludes the offering of specialty courses in a prelicensure curriculum. Thus, many schools of nursing have eliminated clinical rotations on psychiatric units and have addressed mental health concerns in a more cursory manner by subsuming this area of care in other settings, for example, during a community health experience. Not addressing mental health nursing as a distinct entity may, in part, reflect how some faculty are afraid of individuals with mental illness. Students mirror this and often are relieved to be able to opt out of working with "those people." Allowing all Edgewood nursing students the chance to work openly with persons for whom mental illness is at the forefront of care helps them to grapple overtly with such fear, and, on the whole, to overcome it as illustrated by the following student comments.

> I am different as a result of my work in this clinical in many ways. I think that the biggest one is that I have really learned not to judge people by where they live . . . I was really nervous that someone would do something to hurt me or one of my fellow students. I now understand that it is just like anywhere else that people live.

> Before this semester I thought that people with mental illness were all crazy, and walked around acting weird all the time . . . I learned that if you talk to them, they are pretty normal in most instances . . . and they are some nicest people I have ever met. . . . They have the same emotions as people without mental illness and are hurt by the stigma they have to endure.

When entering Edgewood's program many students conceptualize nursing simply as a series of tasks that fulfill medical orders, though a few have a slightly more evolved understanding of it as a career option guaranteeing employment. In NRS 210, students learn about the nurse-patient relationship as a dynamic association between an identified expert (the nurse) and one seeking his or her council to achieve health (the client). They explore the relevance, dynamics, and goals of the relationship, which is assumed to be based on trust and progress through phases. Their interactions with healthy seniors and families in NRS 211 afford them the opportunity to practice vital communication and health assessment skills in a relatively benign atmosphere. In NRS 310-311 they often lose sight of these as they are inundated with the technical knowledge necessary for safe practice on acute inpatient units. Their budding confidence in their mechanical skills when they arrive in NRS

341 is one of the greatest assets and liabilities they bring into the psychosocial-spiritual component of the course. The assurance from past experience that they can carry out care tasks effectively fosters some openness to clients, but by and large, their vision is limited to looking for problems, especially ones that are physical in nature. It is as if their only tool is a hammer, and thus every client concern must be a nail.

By the time they complete NRS 310-311 students recognize nursing as a science, evidenced in part by their ability to cite sound nursing rationales for care provision. They come to NRS 341 enamored with the technology and material trappings of the trade. A third, and indubitably the most complicated aim of the psychosocial-spiritual component of NRS 341, is to help students exceed their empirical ways of knowing and tap into ethical, aesthetic, and personal expressions of caring. That is to say, we want to foster their ability to practice the art of nursing. This hinges on being able to fashion themselves as therapeutic tools and function within the sometimes puzzling and permeable boundaries of professional nurse-client relationships.

Teaching students about therapeutic boundaries is a little like trying to grasp a handful of sand. The tighter they try to hold on, the more the grains of understanding slide through their fingers. Operating outside the comfortable dictates of institutional expectations and routines, where nurse-client relationships are less easily defined, students become increasingly vulnerable to boundary transgressions, both in terms of becoming over-involved and under-involved with their clients. We hope to inspire in our students a clinical mindfulness that recognizes therapeutic boundaries as fine lines and allows them to discern with whom, when, and under what conditions they may be crossed.

While we do think it important for our clinical sites to allow students to develop longer-term relationships, like Katie and Irene's, we agree with Hagerty and Patusky (2003) that assumptions inherent in the nurse-patient relationship as historically described and practiced may not be congruent with current health care environments. The presumed linearity of therapeutic relationships (i.e., that they progress through phases), the beliefs that trust must occur and therapeutic alliances take time, and role expectations that situate nurses and patients as equally invested though differently capable may no longer lend themselves to care provision of acutely ill patients in the face of increased workloads and decreased resources (Hagerty & Patusky, 2003).

In clinical, where students see the same clients for weeks or even a whole semester, the conditions are seemingly ripe for the development of therapeutic relationships in the classic sense. Even so, Hagerty's and Patusky's wisdom applies in our experience of caring for clients with chronic illness in the hospital, long-term care settings, or on their own turf in the community. Their suggestion that alternative approaches need to consider brief but crucial interaction that assumes patient autonomy, choice, and participation (Hagerty & Patusky, 2003, p. 147) is especially apropos when working with clients whose mental illness may be manifested as a tenuous hold on reality, difficulty trusting, and/ or help-rejecting behaviors.

> I know that I have become more patient... the interview didn't go the way I wanted, but I've come to realize that this resident didn't owe me anything. . . . Things do not always go as you had hoped/planned. . . . Some of the things that need to be done shouldn't be done until after you've gotten a better relationship with your resident.

———————

> The main skill that I developed this semester is that of just being there and not having to fix something for the patient. I have always felt the need to do something for patients. . . . The patient I worked with did not need me to do anything for him, and in fact that could have caused him to back slide in his level of independence. What he needed from me was to just be there and listen to him.

Nursing is often referred to as a *helping* profession, and the most frequent reason our students cite for going into nursing is that they want to help people. Pamela often describes new NRS 341 students as "helper junkies," whose wish to fix everything and everyone can inadvertently usurp the autonomy of those they purport to serve. The psychological literature describes their clumsy, misguided attempts to rescue clients as *enabling* and, like many nurses, they could be labeled *codependent.* Contrary to the biomedical model, we do not regard these as pathological conditions, but, rather, as developmental phases in becoming professional caregivers. We applaud our students desire to help. It is evidence of their compassion and potential to engage in acts of justice. We think of it as undisciplined altruism.

> For the first time since being in nursing school, I realized the importance of the emotional/spiritual dimension of health. I didn't understand how much attitude and outlook actually affect physical health. I have a greater sense of acceptance and tolerance for people who are different from myself

and who I once thought I would not be able to connect with. The most important thing I've learned in this regard is that people don't always want to be the ones being helped, they too like to be the helpers sometimes. . . . It makes sense that it is great for building self-esteem and self-worth.

The fourth aim is to promote student understanding of spiritual health and comfort in providing spiritual care. Like many health care professionals, our students are reluctant to grapple with spirituality in the field, in part because it lacks adequate definition, is difficult to quantify or qualify, and is often misconstrued as synonymous with religion. The word "spirit" derives from the Latin *spiritus*, which literally means "to breathe" (Mish, 1989). Originally, it referred to the life principle or to an animating force bestowed by a deity that was sometimes used synonymously with soul. There is a growing emphasis on spiritual health in wellness paradigms used in health education and health promotion programming; "However, the language to understand man's [sic] spiritual nature is in an embryonic stage and thus impedes full understanding of dynamics of the human spirit" (Seaward, 1991, p. 166).

Holistic perspectives like those of Antonovsky (1987) and Greenberg (1995) identified earlier in the chapter consider spiritual health to be a fundamental aspect of wellness. Spiritual health derives from a belief in some unifying force, like nature, scientific laws, or a divinity (Greenberg, 1995) and is characterized by a sense of meaning in life, faith in the way of the universe, and a feeling of unity with others (Banks, cited in Butler, 1997). This latter quality transcends the sense of connection characteristic of the social component of health. It is expressed as a selflessness that is the basis for the development of human qualities such as love, hope, compassion, trust, sacrifice, honesty, and forgiveness (Banks, cited in Butler, 1997). In his review of definitions of spiritual health Bensley (1991) notes a tendency to view the spiritual component as the unifier and coordinator of the other three dimensions of health.

I always felt comfortable with providing care for the psychosocial needs of people, being able to recognize signs of happiness, sadness, depression, or some other mood alteration. It was the spiritual component I needed some help with, because I really never fully understood the definition of spiritual wellness. I always believed it had to be based on religious belief. Since interviewing Joe I have learned that being religious is just one way to express that one has a spirit, but there are many others. It can be based on religion, but it also could be about nature, feeling alive, or accepting yourself for who you are. Spirituality does not have to be expressed through praying or going to church; planting a tree, going for a walk, or helping others in need can express it. And it is very important to ask how someone is doing spiritually, because it is unique to each individual.

What is spiritual about the psychosocial-spiritual component of NRS 341 is apparent in several ways. Significant time is spent exploring with the residents or patients how spirituality is manifested in their lives, and in teaching students how to purposely inquire about this dimension of health.

> I am beginning to feel more and more comfortable talking about spiritual health, in part because I am learning how to ask questions about it. For example, in the interview, even though Jeff didn't say much about his spirituality, I asked specifically if he felt it was a part of wellness. He believes that religion can be narrow, and that the strength of his spirit comes from his friends and his illness, muscular dystrophy. He says you have to look at life from a broader scope and that people shouldn't close themselves and live narrow lives because that is what makes a person unhappy. His purpose in life is to bring humor to all he encounters and by doing so he helps build his own spirit. Humor gives his life meaning, as do his positive attitude, friends, and outdoor hobbies. Jeff gave some excellent advice at the end of the interview, and this was to listen to people with compassion and also to share laughter with those around you.

The preceding quote conveys a change in perspective that commonly occurs among students when they realize that those they are trying to help often possess keen insight and valuable wisdom. In a written summary of the wellness interview just alluded to, the student author noted a shift in her health orientation that is reflected in the nursing diagnoses she felt had relevance:

1. Mobility impairment related to neuromuscular impairment as evidenced by verbal communication of limitations of physical movement.
2. Pain related to physical condition evidenced by verbal communication of pain, alteration in muscle tone, distracting behavior (humor at times as well as frequent movement and readjustment of body).
3. Spiritual well-being: potential for enhancement related to active development of inner self evidenced by resident identifying how his faith helps him cope with disturbed sleep pattern, depression, poor family communication, and lack of support.

The latter diagnosis reflects not only awareness that the spiritual dimension of health is important, but also an appreciation for the potential of chronic illness in one facet of health to catalyze development in another, and that labels (i.e., nursing diagnoses) can be salutogenic in orientation.

A shared characteristic of all the patients and residents we work with in the psychosocial-spiritual component of the course is that they have chronically been on the receiving end of the helping stick. That they are so often the recipients of someone else's altruism is just one factor that puts them at risk for spiritual distress. Residents and patients tell us that turning the tables and letting them be in the helper role for once gives or restores meaning to their lives, thus catalyzing spiritual health. We regard the residents and patients, quite genuinely, as cofaculty. We engage residents and patients in interviews and groups (to be described later) that we hope they find therapeutic. But we are frank that much of the focus of the clinical experience is on student learning and that there are no guarantees of return on patient and resident investments of time and intimate sharing of their stories.

Students enter the housing project or forensic psychiatric unit with a mentality of US (the young, well, strong, and resourceful), and THEM (the old, sick, weak, and poor). Once they get to know the residents and patients, a deep sense of WE emerges. As the residents and students come to see themselves in one another, the students begin questioning whether they are perhaps reaping more benefit from the experience than are the residents or patients. In effect, they transform the adage, "There but for the grace of God go I," to "There, with God's grace, go I."

> I am much more aware of hidden communities. Now when I'm shopping or driving down the street, I notice people more. I wonder where they live and what their community is like. When I see mentally or economically challenged individuals, I wonder what they face in their daily lives and if their needs are being met.
>
> In the past, whenever I would see someone exhibiting symptoms of mental illness while I was riding the bus or walking on the street, I would seek to physically distance myself. . . . I only saw the symptoms, I didn't see the person. I've come to see [a resident] as this very nice, intelligent woman who is struggling to cope with a mental illness. . . . She's a person, like anybody else, who is plagued by symptoms, the same way I would be if I were in her shoes.

> I have always thought of myself as a people person, but I had never before been exposed to people with mental illness. At first, I just wanted to survive

the clinical because I was afraid of the unknown, and now I see these people are not much different from me. We all need the same things: love, family, belonging, a place to call home, and understanding.

Operating outside the comfortable dictates of institutional expectations and routines, where nurse-client relationships are less easily defined, increases student vulnerability to transgressions of therapeutic boundaries. Exploring and caring for a variety of psychosocial and spiritual concerns that can be rather amorphous and ephemeral makes the work of this component of NRS 341 especially difficult. Staying within the confines of professional behavior and maintaining what Pamela sometimes refers to as a stance of *detached concern*, is more feasible when one is part of an effectively functioning group of caregivers. The importance of collaboration is often assumed in health care and yet we have found little useful direction in undergraduate nursing curricula or the relevant literature for promoting teamwork.

Pamela's frequent caution, "The clients are easy, it's coworkers who are tough to deal with" is always met with vigorous students nods. Most of them have at least part-time health care jobs and have tasted the bitterness of workplace gossip and competition, inept employees, and ineffective supervisors. Often situated in inequitable hierarchies and fragmented into shifts, getting along as a nursing staff can be even more taxing than traversing the borders of nurse-client partnerships. Thus, the fifth and final aim of the psychosocial-spiritual component of the course is to allow students to exercise professionalism and esprit de corps by working together on some of the learning assignments described in the following section.

Methods

The course objectives and five psychosocial-spiritual aims are achieved to a large degree through five explicit learning activities:

1. Composing reaction papers to assigned readings.
2. Conducting and witnessing wellness interviews.
3. Designing and leading wellness groups.
4. Active participation in team debriefings focused on planning and critique clinical work.
5. Independent explorations of the psychosocial and spiritual care continuum.

While students are expected to use all the materials from NRS 340 to prepare for each clinical day, there are two additional required texts for the psychosocial-spiritual component of NRS 341. Students write brief reactions to *How Can I Help?* (Dass & Gorman, 1985) and *The Handicapped, Love and Vocation* (Heberlein, 1989). The first book is a classic in the helping fields that aids students in examining their own values, beliefs, and motives for being nurses. The latter book, an autobiographical account of cerebral palsy and being hospitalized multiple times at the psychiatric institution where half of the students are placed, was written and published by a resident in the neighborhood where the other half spend their semester. All of the students meet with the author and have the opportunity to ask him directly about his experience of living life with several highly stigmatized chronic illnesses.

One of our greatest challenges and delights as teachers is to discover with each student ways to rein in his or her benevolent urges in order to develop *"Helpful Being"* (Dass & Gorman, 1985, p. 38). When students can avoid the "dilemma of the diploma," where help becomes equated with know-how and the nurse-client relationship becomes a transaction between one who knows and one who does not (Dass & Gorman, p. 129), they can develop meaningful partnerships with chronically ill clients. When they learn that, "Chances are that if you can't accept help, you can't really give it" (p. 86), their compassion overcomes their helper junkyism. Coming to terms with the fact that no science is exact heightens their tolerance for and forgiveness of the inevitable mistakes that they, their clients, and others make. Because "The inner work, the work on ourselves, is the foundation of all true service" (Dass & Gorman, p. 211) in both chronic illness courses exploration of student feelings about what they are learning, who they are working with, and their own strengths and frailties is every bit as important as mastery of lab values and other *scientific* parameters. As two students put it in their final self-evaluations:

> I think that reading Dass and Gorman has opened my eyes a bit and made me question what my needs are and why I have a desire to help. Is it for personal satisfaction, or praise? This is something I am still trying to figure out, and I think it will be important to revisit this question throughout my career because it may change. Another thing that I have learned this semester is to be more aware of how I am feeling. It is important for me to identify how and why I feel the way I do and try to change the situation or come up with ways to deal with it, such as taking time for myself, deep breathing, and other relaxation techniques.

I believe that the most important thing I have learned in this clinical that will help protect me from burnout is the understanding of the true definition of help. Going into nursing school, we have a stereotype that nurses have to *always* help. That can lead to burnout. I have learned that I can't always fix *everything* or make everything better for someone. We have learned that helping someone does not always mean doing the traditional things we thought it was. It has been important for me to realize that sometimes people just need someone to listen.

The wellness interviews, groups, and debriefings are closely linked and collectively intended to give the students opportunities to practice the skills essential for discerning psychosocial and spiritual health concerns, planning and leading therapeutic groups, and working as effective team members. They also provide a forum for integrating the theory taught in NRS 340 with what the students are doing in NRS 341, as well as a ready means for instructor evaluation of student ability and progress.

During the first half of the semester each student completes at least one wellness interview with a resident or patient. The instructor collaborates with the staff at each site to identify persons who might be willing to help the students learn about wellness and interviewing. These individuals are invited to function as coteachers, and they know that the interviews are confidential and principally to promote student learning. Any benefit to the interviewee is secondary and most often stems from having the chance to be the provider rather than the recipient of help.

Each wellness interview takes about one-half hour, and the subsequent debriefing is a similar length. The instructor and the interviewer's six student-peers are witnesses who document in writing their observations and impressions of the process. Their notes are later given to the interviewer to aid in writing up the interaction. The interviewer has one week to turn in his or her written summary to the instructor along with all the student notes. Thus, the instructor can assess both the work of the interviewer and the witnesses. Table 5.1 gives an overview of the interview process. Two samples of completed summaries can be found in Appendix B.

At the conclusion of the interview, the interviewee is excused and an oral critique ensues. One aspect of the interview debriefing is to collectively identify common client interests and concerns in order to develop meaningful wellness groups for the second half of the semester. Students from all clinical sections do preparatory reading on group

TABLE 5.1 Wellness Interviews

The instructor, in collaboration with staff from the various clinical sites, invites residents or patients to help teach students about wellness and interviewing. The interviewees come willingly and are informed that the interviews are confidential, focused on wellness, and primarily for the purpose of student learning. At the end of each interview, the interviewee is excused, and the students and instructor critique what went on. Each interview takes about one-half hour, and the debriefing is a similar length.

During a given interview, the witnesses are instructed to document their observations and impressions of the process. They receive the note form, which is intended to aid in data collection rather than in prescribing what should or should not be documented. At the conclusion of the interview, the observers give their notes to the interviewer to use in writing up the interview summary.

Client Wellness Interview Notes

Note Taker Name: Name of Interviewer:
Date: Clinical Site:

Client Description   Client Initials:
Gender: Age: Marital Status:

Client Perspective on Wellness
How does the client describe wellness?
Does the client regard himself or herself as well?
Can the client articulate any wellness goals?

Spirit (use spiritual assessment tools as appropriate—available on Blackboard)
1.   Spiritual orientation, traditions, customs
2.   Religious affiliation
3.   Values and beliefs
     What is important in your life?
     What gives your life meaning?

Mind/Mental Status Assessment: Discerned through observation and questioning. Feel free to experiment with any screening tools you would like (see possible tools on Blackboard). Be sure to include any abnormal findings.
1.   General description (appearance, motor activity, speech pattern, general attitude)
2.   Emotions (mood and affect)
3.   Thought process—form and content (observe rate & flow of speech, associations made, logical flow)
4.   Perception
5.   Sensorium and cognition
     a.   Orientation (person, place, time, circumstances)
     b.   Memory (recent, remote, confabulation)

(continued)

TABLE 5.1   *(continued)*

6. Calculation (might use Folstein)
7. Impulse control
8. Judgment and insight
    a.   Ability to solve problems
    b.   Ability to make decisions
    c.   Knowledge about self
    d.   Coping and/or defense mechanisms

Body (Check any of Roy's physiological modes, in which there are concerns or needs, and comment on what they are)

1. Activity & rest: (ambulation, ADL, sleep, energy level)
2. Nutrition (height, weight, diet)
3. Elimination (problems, concerns, recent changes)
4. Oxygenation (smoker?)
5. Fluid and electrolytes
6. Endocrine
7. Protection (any fall risk?)
8. Senses (sight, hearing, pain)
9. Neurological
10. Reproductive (sexuality)

Medication Profile (List *all* medications (PRNs included) the client is currently taking).

Milieu (Psychosocial and Environmental Concerns: DSM IV–Axis IV). Indicate strengths or deficits in the following areas:

1. Primary support group
2. Social environment
3. Education
4. Occupation
5. Housing
6. Economics
7. Access to health care services
8. Interaction with the legal system
9. Other—specify

Nursing Diagnosis: What problems or needs are apparent and how would you label them in nursing terminology?

Interviewer Feedback: What did you learn in watching this interview that you can use to strengthen your ability to do effective interviews?

TABLE 5.1 *(continued)*

After completing an interview and reflecting on his or her peers' notes, the interviewer summarizes the interaction. In light of the limited time available for the interview, it is inevitable that there will be some gaps in the data obtained. A key part of the learning experience is discerning where to focus one's attention and how to learn from the interviewee what is most important to him or her.

Within a week of the interview, the interviewer turns in his or her written summary to the instructor, along with all the student notes. Thus, the instructor can assess both the work of the interviewer and the witnesses. The students have the option of using the note format above to write the summary or of organizing their data and assessments in another fashion, but all summaries must include discussion of what the interviewer learned from the experience. Two samples of interview summaries using different write-up styles can be found in Appendix B.

---

theory and join together to learn about designing and implementing therapeutic groups. Each section then collaborates to develop a written group plan outlining the purpose, rationale, description of the target population, member criteria, guidelines for participation, format and structure, and how the group's value will be evaluated. Attached to the general plan are written overviews for each session composed by the student who will be in charge. These include the behavioral objectives, description of the probable activities, projected benefits of the session, and identification of any special arrangements or materials needed.

During the second half of the semester, each student group runs a wellness group tailored to their particular clientele. There are as many sessions of the group as there are students to lead them (usually seven) and each session is about an hour in duration. As is the case with the wellness interviews, there are several additional written assignments associated with the wellness group. Each student completes a summary of the one session s/he led and a group progress note. At the end of the semester, students from each clinical section cooperatively compose a brief summary of the six sessions of their group. Appendix C provides a copy of the progress note for documenting member participation and samples of a group plan and leadership and group summaries.

Like the interviews, a debriefing follows each wellness group session. In both instances, debriefings help set the tone for teamwork and provide a way to reflect on what is going well and what needs to be improved. Witnessing their peers and instructor in interviews, groups, and debriefings allows students a vicarious view of their own strengths and limits and helps them to develop more productive ways to give and receive constructive feedback. To promote student involvement, the instructor regularly reminds the participants of the confidentially of the debriefings and the importance of maintaining a nonjudgmental attitude.

Each debriefing is characterized by a similar pattern of first giving the identified student (whether in the role of interviewer or group leader) a chance to comment on how she or he felt the experience went. The instructor inquires whether input from others is desired, and if so, what particular kind of feedback is sought. With permission (which so far has been universal), students identify what they learned by observing the interview or group session that can be used to enhance their own work, offer suggestions for alternative approaches, and reinforce what they noted that the interviewer or group leader was doing to advance desired outcomes.

A common theme in the debriefings is how much it means to the students to have an opportunity to watch the instructor and their peers in action. Though many students report feeling anxious when being witnessed, in retrospect they are unanimous in their assessment that any discomfort experienced is greatly outweighed by the benefit of getting constructive input on both their strengths and areas for improvement. Many students comment as well that engaging in the process also seems to evoke empathy for their peers, which results in greater cohesion in the student team.

> I got to experience things I would never have experienced. I'm really glad we had to complete wellness interviews in front of the rest of the class. Even though I was nervous, it really helped me realize what I needed help with and what I already did well. Also, the rest of the group was able to get ideas from the person conducting the interview.

> I can't say I really liked doing the interview. I was very nervous, but I learned a lot in the process. It was good to have you [the instructor] and my friends point out some things I did well that I didn't realize.

> It is so important to get everyone involved with the groups. I felt that because we all worked together on each of the groups, we did better within each of

the sessions. I thought it was an especially valuable experience to have the instructor and peers critique each others work.

The final learning activity involves students in 8 hours of individually negotiated independent visitations to local programs and agencies that provide a variety of psychosocial and spiritually focused services. The assignment exposes them to the continuum of care essential for people living lives with chronic illnesses—especially illnesses that manifest in the mental, social, and spiritual aspects of health. It also gives them an opportunity to learn about psychiatric nursing as a specialty, as the contact person for the visit is often practicing in this capacity.

Students can choose from a list of approved activities or negotiate another experience with the instructor if they have access to relevant opportunities. Examples of possible experiences include but are not limited to visits to local mental heath centers and their affiliated programs, psychiatric inpatient units, meal programs and shelters serving the population of concern, a variety of AA, Al-Anon, and National Alliance for the Mentally Ill sponsored therapeutic groups, and various crisis support programs. Students who are based in the community for the psychosocial-spiritual component are required to spend at least 4 hours of their independent experience time in an inpatient setting, and those based in an inpatient setting are required to spend a minimum of 4 hours in a community-based program.

One student's comment in a course evaluation—"I really enjoyed the independent experiences. I got to get out into the community and do things that I'm interested in."—conveys a common reaction students have to the assignment. Most seem to appreciate the chance to do some exploration on their own. Students write a summary of each experience following the guidelines contained in Table 5.2. Included in the write-ups is discussion of what the student learned that could enhance his/her ability to provide psychosocial and spiritual care to people living with a chronic illness. What stands out for many students is how these experiences alter stereotypes they had of people with mental illness, as was the case with one who visited an AA meeting.

I want to start by saying I absolutely loved the experience, and I will be going again next week so I can do some comparison of two meetings. I guess I loved it so much because it wasn't anything as I expected it to be. I also have to admit that I went thinking I wasn't going to learn much at all because I don't have an alcohol problem. Wow, was I wrong! I learned that these individuals are so courageous. Listening to them made it clear that they want to change, but this is a disease and they just can't snap their fingers and quit.

TABLE 5.2   Independent Experience Guidelines

Student: **Date:**

General Directions

Due: ASAP after you complete the independent experience(s). **Final deadline** _____. After completing your visit(s), respond in writing to each category below and forward your summary to the course instructors. **Take the following outline along** with you as a guide to the information you need for the summary.

Summary Guide for Community-Based Program Visits

Note: When two or more students visit a program together, they may collaborate to write up one summary for that portion of the Independent Experience. Be sure to include all student names on the summary and to notify both instructors if the students are in different sections.

Describe your visit:

1.   Name(s) and location(s) of the program(s)
2.   Date you went and amount of time you spent there
3.   Briefly summarize the activities you were involved in while visiting the program(s)

Program description—for each program you visit indicate the following:

1.   Primary purpose of the program (e.g., housing, meals, vocational assistance, inpatient unit, etc.). Ask staff if there is a mission statement and/or specific program goals
2.   Services provided by the program—what kinds of problems are addressed and how are they addressed? (Note: if you visit Elder Care, please comment on how activities are planned throughout the day to manage the milieu)
3.   How the program is funded (i.e., public or private funds, do the clients pay for services?, etc.)

Client population:

1.   List the criteria for receiving services (i.e. Who can use the program?)
2.   How many clients does the program serve?
3.   Briefly convey any observations you made about the clients who were present at the time you visited

Provider information:

1.   Who are the providers (nurses, social workers, psychologists, psychiatrists, etc.)?
2.   Ask the providers:
     a.   What their primary responsibilities are
     b.   What they find most rewarding about their work
     c.   What they find most difficult about their work

TABLE 5.2   *(continued)*

Student reactions:

1. What did you learn in the visit(s) that will enhance your ability to provide psychosocial-spiritual care to individuals facing chronic illness?
2. Identify any insights or questions the visit(s) evoked for you.

Summary Guide for Inpatient Visits

Identify the unit(s) you visited:

Activity Summary: Write a brief summary of the activities you were involved in during the day.

Client Population:

1. Identify the general characteristics of the population served (report what you observe and what the staff tells you).
2. Describe some of the symptoms of mental illness you saw in evidence.
3. Write up a *very brief* mental status exam for one client you observed and/or spent time with.
    a. General description
    b. Emotions
    c. Thought
    d. Perception
    e. Sensorium and Cognition
    f. Impulse Control
    g. Judgment and Insight

Psychiatric Nursing Roles: Ask as many nurses as possible what they see as their primary responsibilities, and what they like most and least about their work. List responses.

Summary Guides for—

Therapeutic Groups: Identify the name of the group, where it is located, and when you went, then summarize the experience by discussing the following group characteristics.

1. Structure—describe the parameters of the group (e.g., member criteria, open or closed, etc.)?
2. What is the purpose of the group?
3. What are the goals of the group?
4. Identify some of the roles that were apparent, and provide examples of member behaviors that helped you to ascertain them
5. Give some examples of group norms
6. Which of Yalom's therapeutic factors were apparent in the group? Give examples of group occurrences that support your contention that they were present

(continued)

TABLE 5.2   *(continued)*

Educational Presentations—identify the following:

1. Title of the presentation and name of presenter (including credentials)
2. Date, time, and place of presentation
3. Brief summary of the key points
4. What you learned from the presentation that will enhance your ability to provide psychosocial and spiritual care to people living with a chronic illness

Interviews—identify the following:

1. Date, time, and place of interview
2. Who you interviewed including their credentials and where they work
3. The individual's primary work responsibilities
4. What she or he likes most and least about his or her work
5. What you learned from the interview that will enhance your ability to provide psychosocial and spiritual care to people living with a chronic illness

So how all of this can enhance my ability to provide care really comes down to trying to understand what they are going through and to show some empathy. And don't be stereotypical and think only the "bums" off the street are the ones with an alcoholic problem. Also, don't give up on them if they tell you they can't quit at this time. Don't think that they are a hopeless cause and have no will power. Plenty of the individuals stated last night that it took them many times to quit to finally get to the place they are at now. Plus, I realized last night that spirituality is what get a lot of them through the rough days. Now, if I'm caring for people who have a drinking problem, I will pay attention to their spirit as much as their bodies.

MEDICAL-SURGICAL COMPONENT

As discussed previously, clinical site selection for the medical/surgical component of the course is crucial in achieving the course objectives. Currently, faculty utilize two acute rehab units, one situated in a university hospital, the other in a large not-for-profit facility in the same city. We also make use of subacute units in long-term care facilities, however the lack of consistent RN role models makes utilization of these sites more challenging. More recently, faculty expanded their clinical site selection to include hospice care, incorporating both inpatient care and home care. What becomes paramount in site selection for this component of NRS 341 is that students have opportunities to work with clients and families over an extended period of time. Shortened hospitalizations makes this very difficult and continues to be our biggest challenge in finding appropriate clinical sites.

The clinical course objectives are referenced earlier in this chapter. What follows is an overview of the clinical activities and assignments the students in the med/surg component of this clinical complete to fulfill the course requirements during their 16 weeks. In essence, this is "what we do." Despite the fact that five sections of this portion of clinical run concurrently, faculty members maintain strong communication amongst themselves to ensure continuity between sections while preserving faculty autonomy over their clinical sections and assignments. You might say that 'what we do' is somewhat unified; however, 'how we do it' remains highly individualized.

In many ways, our approach to clinical teaching is rather traditional. Faculty post clinical assignments one to 2 days prior to clinical and are on site throughout the duration of the students 8-hour clinical day. It is the expectation that students prepare for clinical prior to arriving on site for their clinical day by reading the patient or client's record, familiarizing themselves with the medical diagnosis, understanding the client's pharmacological regime and developing their nursing plan of care.

What transpires in a typical clinical day may appear somewhat uneventful and disappointingly similar to other clinical experiences regardless of the site. Students have ample opportunities to provide physical care, complete physical assessments, pass medications, complete treatments, improve their organizational skills, tape report, document and interact with other staff; these are all very routine activities. In the end, what is different is the development and implementation of a cognitive structure that embraces whole-person care.

Kelly's Thank You

About 10 weeks into our first semester at Hospice, one of my students, Kelly, approached me requesting to care for Dan in room 1. She proceeded to tell me that she had cared for Dan during her last clinical while she was in acute care. Dan had just been diagnosed with a terminal disease. In addition, just months prior to his diagnosis, Dan had lost his wife. Their only son, Tom, was single with minimal support systems to help him during this difficult time.

Apparently, Dan had given the nurses a hard time while hospitalized elsewhere, and when the hospice nurses first realized I had assigned him to

Kelly, they expressed concern that perhaps this might not be an appropriate assignment for a student nurse. Dan was angry about his diagnosis and his wife's death, and he made sure everyone knew it. The staff thought that a student shouldn't have to deal with someone like Dan. I, on the other hand, consider most challenging situations appropriate for students. Dan remembered Kelly and agreed to have her care for him when I asked him. Tom also remembered Kelly and was pleased that she would be caring for his Dad.

Kelly's first clinical day with Dan proceeded without any difficulties—or so I thought. However, the next day, I received a phone message from hospice, asking me to call regarding the student that cared for Dan. My heart sank. My first thoughts centered on medication errors or other problems. I knew Dan was very angry about his situation. Perhaps his interactions with Kelly weren't as positive as I had thought and he had voiced some complaints about his care.

I called the center immediately and spoke with the case manager. She informed me that both Dan and Tom were requesting that Kelly continue to care for Dan throughout the rest of his stay. She further informed me that, "She was the only one Dan could get along with," and she asked, "Would she please continue working with them?" I agreed. Unfortunately, Dan passed away the day before we returned for our next clinical. Kelly never had another chance to care for Dan.

Two days later, another student saw Dan's obituary in the local paper. She called Kelly to read it to her. Toward the end of Dan's obituary, after thanking the hospice staff for the care he received, he added, "and a special thank you to the Edgewood College nursing students, especially Kelly." Kelly was so astonished, she cried.

I later asked Kelly to reflect on her thoughts and feelings about the entire experience. Here, a man with 65 years of experiences fondly remembers and thanks a student nurse who cared for him for 16 hours of those 65 years. Kelly said, "It was OK with me that he was angry. I just let him be him."

Here, a student successfully demonstrates her ability to incorporate a cognitive structure that embraces whole-person care into her nursing practice. One that respects a dying man's anger and "lets him be him."

Looking Beyond the Present

Providing care for the future, in part, addresses overcoming the deficit model put forth by nursing diagnosis. Nursing diagnoses, as part of the nursing process, can perpetuate a deficit mind-set that fails to capture client and family strengths and may be shortsighted when applied to chronic illness management and living a life. Despite its limitations, students in their previous semester of acute care utilize nursing process, along with nursing diagnosis, as a framework for assessing, planning, intervening, and evaluating. In their previous semester, students used a systems approach to problem identification and care planning. Each week students concentrated on one element from Roy's adaptation model, such as nutrition, mobility, circulation, or elimination to direct their implementation of the nursing process.

In the clinical course, one of our goals is aimed at progressing student thinking from collecting data on one body system to a more inclusive, whole person assessment along with the consideration of client and family health. Nursing diagnoses are supplemented with identification of client/family strengths. Each week, students are challenged to identify health in the context of a medical diagnosis that suggests illness, even death and dying. Nursing interventions are identified based on client strengths. Regardless of what type of paperwork each instructor requires on a weekly basis, students must assess health in the context of whole-person care, and this assessment must be reflected in their nursing interventions and nursing care.

Decisions That Reflect Context

One very important component of this clinical is exposing students to the entire spectrum of care. This can be achieved at our various sites in a number of ways. Students at the hospice site not only provide care in the acute inpatient unit, they also spend time with staff from the in-home team, making home visits. Students also work with nurses on the admission team, seeing clients as they enter hospice care and interacting with the case manager on the inpatient unit. These experiences serve to provide exposure to the continuum of care at this site.

Students in the acute rehab settings, likewise, have opportunities to experience the entire spectrum of rehab care by spending time on the acute neurological intermediate care (IMC) unit, where clients frequently receive their initial care following stroke or head injury. Students can also continue to work with their clients and families post discharge in the day-rehab program, an outpatient program for clients who require further rehab services. Opportunities are also available for students to participate with other team members, going on home visits prior to discharge or to attending recreational outings, such as dining out, to assess for any unforeseen issues in preparation for discharge.

These opportunities are not implemented as observational experiences: Students do not go to watch someone else work. Rather, they actively participate in all aspects of nursing care, ranging from physical care to discharge planning, writing referrals, or contacting other agencies. Following these experiences, students complete written assignments integrating their nursing assessments with discharge planning and reflecting on and integrating whole-person care.

This exposure to the entire spectrum of care is vital for students as they develop decision-making skills that reflect context—that is, living a life with a chronic illness and whole-person care. The opportunity to hypothetically refocus their lens from close-up to panoramic is clearly reflected in students' daily functioning in their med/surg sites. As stated earlier, what the students do during their 8-hour clinical is not that different from their previous semester. What is dramatically different, however, is their thinking and the larger context they are able to reference in making appropriate clinical decisions. The following story demonstrates this process.

Harry's Discharge

Harry was a 72-year-old gentleman who suffered a left sided cerebral vascular accident (CVA). As Harry prepared for discharge, it appeared likely that one of his discharge medications would include warfarin. While in the hospital, Harry's blood work was drawn on a daily basis, medication orders were written, and the nursing staff dispensed the exact dose—a fairly uncomplicated process. Plans were being made for Harry to have his blood work done twice a week after discharge. He would then follow up by phoning his local physician for the results. Harry was to be sent home with 2-mg, 5-mg, and 10-mg tablets of warfarin, along with directions similar to a sliding scale for insulin. Based on the results of his blood work and the dosage scale, it was postulated that Harry would figure out what combination of tablets he needed to take to achieve the desired dose. While this may seem like a feasible plan while in the hospital, the nursing student was familiar with issues related to transportation for blood work or arranging for in-home blood draws, phoning physician's offices, obtaining laboratory results over the phone, and inaccurate dosage calculations. After discussing the feasibility of this plan with members of the health team, the decision was made for an alternate medication.

What the students do in the clinical course is not that different from the previous semester. What transforms is their thinking, informed by a richer whole-person context. This transformative thinking is vital, as the majority of our students will seek employment in acute-care settings initially upon graduation. We hope that this transformative thinking will continue to inform their nursing practice regardless of their employment setting.

Providing Care for the Future

One important facet in providing care for the future includes the development of partnerships with clients and families. Developing and understanding the role of the nurse as a patient and family advocate is predicated on the ability to form partnerships in care, such as the partnership described earlier in this chapter, between Irene and the student nurse Katie. Establishing partnerships serves as a prelude for nurses when advocating for client's and family's future care needs.

To this end, ensuring that students care for the same clients throughout the duration of their hospitalization becomes paramount. Even though students are on site only 1 day per week, most students have the opportunity to care for their clients at least two or three times, sometimes longer. Faculty at all of our clinical sites appreciate the significance of this continuity; in fact, it is the driving force behind our site selection and continues to present our biggest challenge as our enrollment increases.

A second imperative component in providing care for the future includes the development of partnerships within the health care team. To this end, all our clinical sites provide opportunities for students to become actively involved in interdisciplinary group meetings. At hospice, inter-disciplinary group (IDG) meets the day before the students are on site. Student attendance is mandatory. While multidisciplinary group meetings serve several important functions, it is the student's presence that opens the door to their integration into the team. Initially, the transition from looking beyond the present to providing care for the future can be somewhat turbulent, as reflected in this story:

Colleen's Reality Check

This was our first semester at the hospice center in our city. Prior to the start of the semester, staff members strongly encouraged me to have our students attend the interdisciplinary group meetings held on Wednesday. Members in attendance include nursing staff, physicians, bereavement counselors, social workers, chaplains, pharmacists, nutritionists, and dietary personnel, to name a few. On our first day, we were all introduced and properly welcomed. Everyone was very kind and genuinely pleased to have the nursing students on site. My entire clinical group listened attentively for 2 hours while each client was discussed, attempting to feign interest. Not knowing any of these individuals, it was difficult to appreciate the relevance of the conversation. I, on the other hand, was convinced that the students would be ecstatic about this chance to see the entire team working together like a well-oiled machine, solving every clinical problem that was brought forth in a beautifully orchestrated demonstration of teamwork. My high-on-life teaching moment was short lived: The bubble burst prematurely when, at the end of the conference, a student disappointedly remarked to me, "But I still don't know if my patient needs a bath tomorrow."

While students enter this clinical focused on the solitary role of providing physical care for individuals at the bedside, this portion of the course offers students their first encounter with collaborative practice. The nurse as a team member takes on a tangible role that previously exceeded the student's limited scope of practice. Student participation as an involved team member is a course expectation. Throughout the semester, students are able to develop their skill and confidence in this role and find their voice in articulating patient and family information in a team setting.

Assignments

As previously discussed, preserving faculty autonomy over their clinical sections and assignments is extremely important. While what we do is somewhat unified, how we do it remains highly individualized and is determined, in part, by the uniqueness of each clinical site.

Care Planning

The first clinical objective for this course addresses the application of the nursing process to maximize clients' functioning with chronic illness. To this end, each faculty has formulated its own tool (referred to as the data collection tool, overview of care form, or daily worksheet) to facilitate student data collection and care planning. The purpose of these written assignments is to evaluate critical thinking in the context of nursing process and care planning. Similarly, worksheets for medication management have been developed to reflect the individual student needs at each agency. Remembering that our clinical sites are either rehab, subacute, or hospice, the primary emphasis is not acute management of primary disorders. Despite this, students have ample opportunity to work with clients experiencing a number of chronic illnesses such as hypertension, diabetes, chronic obstructive pulmonary disorder (COPD), depression, or anxiety, to name a few.

Instructors individually determine how this information is best collected, evaluated, and returned to students. In addition, the frequency of these assignments is also individually determined, based on mastery of the process. Our goal is twofold: First, we want students to be able to complete a holistic assessment on a client, formulate and document their plan of care, implement or delegate the provision of care, and evaluate the care provided. Second, we hope that our students are beginning to develop the knowledge base required to demonstrate anticipatory thinking—that is, consideration of the numerous potential problems nurses deal with on a daily basis. Recognition or consideration of potential problems directly impacts our nursing care. For example, if a client is receiving insulin therapy, "at risk for hypoglycemia related to insulin therapy" should be included in the client's problem list as formulated by the student. Similarly, if a client is receiving opioid analgesia, "at risk for alteration in bowel function/constipation" should be addressed. Helping students advance their expertise by identifying potential problems also helps them develop insight into preventive interventions, which ultimately enhances their capacity to 'think like a nurse'. Tables 5.3 and 5.4 provide examples of care planning sheets and data collection instruments that the students use.

Medication Management

Clinical faculty in this component of the course also have their students complete a variety of medication quizzes throughout the semester. De-

TABLE 5.3 Nursing Care Plan

Nursing Diagnosis	Goal	Nursing Interventions & Rationale	Outcome of Interventions	Evaluation of Goal

TABLE 5.4   Daily Worksheet

Date: _____

Room: _____ Name (initials only): _____ Student: _____
Allergies: _____

Admit diagnosis: PMH:

From report: (include info from   Giving report:
Wed. team mtg.)

Responsibilities to complete: MISC:

                                         _____ Discharge Planning needs

                                         _____ Psycho-social spiritual needs

                                         _____ Family needs

---

signed to focus on clinical pharmacology unique to each unit, these quizzes serve to evaluate student's retention and application of content previously studied in their pharmacology class. Some of these quizzes are short 10-point exams on topics such as anticoagulants, diuretics, or antihypertensive medications. Other quizzes are more inclusive, addressing a larger spectrum of drug classifications and appropriate laboratory values to monitor during therapy. Table 5.5 provides a sample medication worksheet.

Teaching Project

Students also complete a teaching/learning project in this portion of their clinical. Building on the knowledge gained regarding group pro-

TABLE 5.5   Medication Sheet

Medication & Class	Dose	Route	Time	Mech. of Action	Purpose	Side Effects (NI)	Labs to Monitor

cess in their companion component of this class, students are required to complete a teaching/learning project for a group of individuals. Previously, students in acute care completed a teaching/learning project for an individual. This might include discharge instructions, medication instructions or wound care instructions. In this course, students are challenged to assess, plan, intervene, and evaluate their teaching for a group.

One semester, students spent 4 hours each week at Elder Care of Dane County. This organization provides a multitude of services for the underserved senior citizens in the area. One service includes in-home assistance with ADL's. Provided mostly by nursing assistants or unlicensed assistive personnel, this group expressed an interest in learning more about diabetes—specifically, what it is, when to give sugar, why is foot care so important, what is insulin, and other basic concepts. The student nurse group divided the topic into sections such as medications, diet, foot care, exercise, complications, and pathophysiology. Each student prepared a brief discussion on each topic, keeping in mind the intended audience. To make the activity more fun and meaningful, following the presentations, students divided the group into two teams to play Diabetes Jeopardy. Each topic presented had its own jeopardy category. This 45-minute activity was a huge success, and the personnel attending earned mandatory educational credits required for their continued employment.

Another teaching/learning project requirement that exemplifies clinical partnerships was the student production of an educational video entitled, "Caring for a Patient with a Chest Tube." Students on an acute rehab unit were seeing clients appear on the unit earlier and earlier in their recovery. Staff nurses on rehab were not accustomed to patients with chest tubes, hence the need for the development and production of the video. Students researched the topic, wrote the script, and produced the video, which will be used by all the rehab staff as an educational resource tool for semesters to come.

Although the nature of the project can vary from between clinical sites, three basic requirements remain constant: (1) the project topic/idea must evolve from problems or needs identified by the staff, (2) the project must involve utilization of the nursing process for a group, and (3) there must be a concrete end product developed that is left with the agency for future educational use. The teaching/learning project is an opportunity for students to give back to the agency and strengthen our clinical partnerships. Table 5.6 presents the guidelines for this assignment.

STUDENT ASSESSMENT

Teaching and learning involve student and instructor in a relationship of mutual accountability. "By accountability we mean that the teacher is responsible to teach what he has promised learners will learn. And the learners are responsible to do the work of learning" (Vella, 2002, p. 213). Developing human potential is a core function of higher education and involves both a process and a holistic set of desired outcomes. The process is reflected in the ability to function in increasingly complex and refined ways, and the set of outcomes encompasses a host of desirable skills, knowledge, competencies, beliefs, and attitudes (Kuh, Gonyea, & Rodriguez, 2002, pp. 100–101). Nursing education directs student development in such manner as to maximize not only the potential of the student but also those that she or he will serve. These goals that potentially the clinical course seeks to develop are embodied in the six

TABLE 5.6   Guidelines for Client Teaching/Learning Project

Objectives:

1. Utilize the nursing process as teacher in a clinical situation
2. Develop a teaching/learning plan based on assessment of the learner and teaching/learning principles
3. Integrate knowledge of specific health content with awareness of factors that influence learning
4. Incorporate learner outcomes in the plan for evaluation of teaching

Directions:

1. Prior to preparing the teaching session,
   a. Select a clinical learning situation. This session is designed to increase your ability to teach a group of individuals. Examples include teaching a group of CNAs, RNs, LPNs, patients, families, etc.
   b. Plan with clinical faculty for the specific teaching project. Selecting a topic is best accomplished by asking the intended audience for suggestions regarding a topic or topics of their choice
   c. Clinical instructor will review the teaching plan prior to implementation
   d. Students can work in groups or present individually. (This decision will be made by the clinical instructor based on the units needs)
2. Prepare teaching plan (utilizing steps of the nursing process) to meet the group's learning needs
   a. Assess the learner. Include the following:
      i. learner's status: developmental status, cognitive level, psychomotor skills, affective status
      ii. learner's priorities: is this information something the learner wants to know or something you think he or she should know?
      iii. learner's current knowledge, skills
      iv. learner's available resources
      v. learner's readiness to learn
      vi. other pertinent data: what have your learners prior experiences been with the topic being presented, and are there any negative images you may want to consider?
   b. Assess your level of expertise
   c. Develop a teaching/learning plan, including the following:
      i. learner outcomes
      ii. specific content of plan(in outline form): clear and appropriate
      iii. teaching strategies selected and rationale
   d. Implement the plan, describing preparation of learner, time allocation, context of teaching/learning situation
   e. Evaluate achievement of client outcomes, client's response, and self-evaluation as a teacher. Evaluation is achieved by completing some form of a pre/post test. This does not necessarily need to be a written test, but can be included as part of the teaching session
3. Clinical faculty will discuss all components of the teaching/learning project with students throughout the planning, implementation, and evaluation process

course objectives. But how do we know that these goals have been realized?

"How do they know they know? We believe an accountable response is, Because they did it!" (Vella, 1998, p. xi). The clinical course is graded on a pass/fail basis that sets safe practice as the bottom line for determining progression to the next level of study. When our students apply nursing process to maximize client functioning, advocate for needed resources to assure continuity of care, collaborate with multidisciplinary teams to promote client participation in treatment, demonstrate commitment and accountability for clinical decision-making, develop themselves as therapeutic agents while maintaining respect for client individuality, and make clinical decisions that reflect consideration of context we are confident in that they will "do no harm" and can advance to the next level of courses (NRS 410-411).

As an aid to the assessment process we have operationalized the course objectives as critical behaviors that must be demonstrated in order to pass the course. These are contained in the Clinical Evaluation Tool (CET) for each component of the course, which appears in Appendix D. The student must receive a satisfactory or better rating for each expected behavior on both CETs, as well as satisfactory ratings for all required assignments, in order to receive a passing grade for the course.

The instructor enters evaluative comments on the CET and shares these with the student throughout the semester in order to emphasis what she or he is doing well and what needs work. Students have conveyed that putting such feedback in writing makes a far greater impact than simply conveying it verbally. Each student meets with his/her instructors from both the medical-surgical and psychosocial-spiritual components of the course in individual midterm and final evaluation conferences.

"The way we diagnose our students' condition will determine the kind of remedy we offer" (Palmer, 1998, p. 41). We assume that students "come with both experience and personal perceptions of the world based on that experience and all deserve respect as subjects of a learning dialogue" (Vella, 2002, p. 27). Thus, we expect our students to be collaborators in evaluating their performance as it relates to the learning objectives. We engage in an educational dialogue that recognizes self-assessment as an essential skill for safe clinical practice.

We teach students to critically exam their own strengths and areas for development, as well as those of their clients, peers, and instructors. This is done formally by having students write summaries of their accomplishments at midterm and at the end of the course, as illustrated in the sample CETs in Appendix E. In addition, many of the written assignments include a reflective component that has students appraise what they learned from the experience being summarized. The student comments found in the section of this chapter describing the psychoso-cial-spiritual component of the course are illustrative of this.

More informal formative assessment occurs each clinical day as students and instructors gather to question what was learned and accomplished, what was useful, and what needs to change. Students are expected to continually discern how their thinking and behavior reflects their professional formation. Just one example of this is the tradition of inquiring toward the close of each interview or group debriefing session in the psychosocial component of the course, "How was what we did today *nursing?*"

One approach to knowing about student learning is embodied in a positive or scientific view of education, while another relies on more subjectivist and intuitionist premises (Gray, 2002). We employ both. The first is evidenced in the fact that we specify in advance overt expectations (i.e., course objectives) that are translated into student outcomes (i.e., professional behaviors), which are directly observed and documented on the CET. The latter assessment method, though not as explicit, is by no means less important. Assuming that "goals will come first and action comes later is frequently radically wrong. Human choice behavior is at least as much a process for discovering goals as for acting on them" (Cohen & March, 1991, cited in Gray, 2002, p. 53). Throughout and at the conclusion of each semester, students express verbally and in writing how they are different as a result of the work they do in the clinical course. Inevitably, and most fortunately, "What learners learn is much beyond what the teachers plan" (Vella, 2002, p. 26) and we are frequently surprised and delighted by the immeasurable depth of the transformation students describe.

I learned a lot about myself as a person from this clinical. I learned the importance of not labeling people with a disability as the disability itself . . . of setting boundaries, not only in my professional life but also in my personal life . . . of being prepared and being confident . . . and that it's ok to ask for help. I so didn't want to feel like I didn't know what I was doing or that I couldn't handle the experience, but I learned that my teammates are there to help me, and that they might have similar questions or even learn from my experiences/mistakes. It's so important to collaborate and stand by each other . . . [and] maintain healthy relationships and a rewarding life outside of school, because you can't be good to others when you're not good to yourself.

REFERENCES

American Psychiatric Association. (1994). *Diagnostic and statistical manual of mental disorders* (4rd ed.). Washington, DC: American Psychiatric Association.

Antonovsky, A. (1987). *Unraveling the mystery of health: How people manage stress and stay well.* San Francisco: Jossey-Bass.

Bensley, R. J. (1991). Defining spiritual health: A review of the literature. *Journal of Health Education, 22*(5), 287–290.

Butler, J. T. (1997). *Principles of health education and health promotion* (2nd ed.). Englewood, CO: Morton Publishing.

Dass, R., & Gorman, P. (1985). *How can I help?* New York: Alfred A. Knopf.

Gray, P. J. (2002). The roots of assessment. In T. W. Banta (Ed.), *Building a scholarship of assessment* (pp. 49–66). San Francisco: Jossey-Bass.

Greenberg, J. S. (1995). Health education clarified. In J. S. Greenberg, *Health education* (pp. 2–14). Madison, WI: Brown & Benchmark Publishers.

Hagerty, B. M., & Patusky, K. L. (2003). Reconceptualizing the nurse-patient relationship. *Journal of Nursing Scholarship, Second Quarter,* 145–150.

Heberlein, A. (1989). *The handicapped, love and vocation.* Madison, WI: Heberlein, A.

Kuh, G. D., Gonyea, R. B., & Rodriguez, D. P. (2002). The scholarly assessment of student development. In T. W. Banta (Ed.), *Building a scholarship of assessment* (pp. 100–127). San Francisco: Jossey-Bass.

Mish, F. C. (Ed.) (1989). *Merriam Webster's word histories.* Springfield, MA: Merriam-Webster, Inc.

Palmer, P. (1998). *The courage to teach.* San Francisco: Jossey-Bass.

Seaward, B. L. (1991). Spiritual wellbeing: A health education model. *Journal of Health Education, 22*(3), 16.

Vella, J. (1998). *How do they know they know?* San Francisco: Jossey-Bass.

Vella, J. (2002). *Learning to listen, learning to teach: The power of dialogue in educating adults.* San Francisco: Jossey-Bass.

6

Using the Experiences of Students

When a person is healthy and whole, the head and the heart are both-and, not either-or, and teaching that honors that paradox can help make us all more whole. (Palmer, 1998, p. 64)

Chapters 4 and 5 discussed our approach to teaching both didactic and clinical content, founded on the themes presented in chapter 3. This final chapter, somewhat allegorically, completes the teaching circle. As part of integrating the college values into our teaching and course work, we invite three former students to return as guest speakers—*content* experts, if you will. Initially, two of these three were still undergraduates when they began teaching with us. Chapter 4 briefly addressed the value of having students serve in the role of instructor. It is not only the highly personal and complementary nature of what they present below that inspires us as teachers. Witnessing the professionalism of our previous students as they astutely and clearly articulate where the knowledge and skills they gleaned from the chronic illness courses has taken them is immensely rewarding. Their stories attest to the fact that this partnership has also been intensely meaningful for them.

Greg's Story

We first met Greg as an undergraduate student in our nursing program. Greg was a reentry student, having withdrawn from the program several years earlier. Though about 10 years older than the more traditional undergraduate student and somewhat of a loner, Greg was an eager learner. He embraced each clinical or classroom situation as an opportunity to expand his knowledge and skills. While some students unintentionally sabotage their own learning with comments such as, "What has

133

this got to do with Nursing?" Greg was always open to every client/ student encounter and could envision the nursing role in an assortment of circumstances. In addition, Greg was beginning to appreciate the significance of process, not just outcomes. What none of us knew then, though some of us suspected, was that Greg had an addiction.

Greg graduated from our program and worked out of state for about 3 years before things got complicated. His specialty area is oncology, viewed as a daily dose of pain and suffering with ample access to narcotics. After approximately 18 months in mandatory rehab, Greg began working again. Initially, his license was restricted in that he could not pass narcotics. It was during this time, however, that he found he could assist his fellow staff nurses by starting their IVs for them while they passed his narcotics. Consequently, he wasn't a liability but instead rapidly developed into a valuable asset by becoming one of the best IV nurses on the unit. When Greg reveals this story with our undergraduates, he talks about how he chooses not to sit in a chair next to the bed when starting IVs; instead, Greg kneels down on one knee. He discloses how he draws on the brief 5 or 10 seconds prior to IV insertion to clandestinely recite his own simple prayer, asking that his talents be made available to help him assist this patient as he completes this sometimes painful procedure. We know about this personal practice, because twice a year, Greg spends 2 hours with the NRS 340 class sharing his own lived experience. Each class is somewhat different, but every class is equally as compelling and riveting.

Greg's participation in the theory course as a guest speaker has meaning on three different levels. His poignant account of his personal and professional struggles evokes strong feelings in the students. For some, it is an awareness of their own potential vulnerability as nurses. Others are offended by what they perceive as a lack of morale fiber, or search for solutions to *fix* Greg. All are left with a better grasp on what it means to live a life with a chronic illness, especially one that is highly stigmatized. Collaborating with Greg as a student-turned-colleague gives NRS 340 faculty a chance to actualize the Edgewood College value of partnership on a functional level. For Greg, teaching our class presents an assortment of challenges and has, over the past semesters, helped create meaning in his life. From this, he has cultivated a desire to continue his education to become a teacher. He writes about the meaning of first being a NRS 340 student and then shifting to the role of teacher.

I was told, early in my college career, that education had nothing to do with learning. I agreed with that statement not out of some enlightened higher conscience but because it sounded cool and the professor scared me to death. Professional Nursing: Long-term Health Issues (NRS 340) reinforced this notion and served as a springboard to a more enlightened point of view.

I arrived in NRS 340 with all the prejudices of a want-to-be nurse, ready to shape the world in my image and thus really heal those who wanted to be healed. Prior to this class, I had never paid much attention to the fact that the people who entrusted their lives, or the lives of their loved ones, to me came attached to families, to friends, and to their own life experiences and views. This was really quite a revelation to me. It was also pointed out to my classmates and me that the time I would spend with them was, by comparison, one of the many grains of sand in the hourglass of their life. My interest was immediately piqued. Over the next several months, I found myself in the company of two very dedicated and gifted teachers. The lectures were often interactive, employing case files, role-playing and story telling. The conventions of teaching and learning were shelved for now, and I was challenged to apply theory to real life. This new approach—critical thinking, if you will—was stimulating, vexing, wonderful, and a huge pain—all at the same time. The comprehensive take-home exams fostered this new skill of critical thinking and gently nudged me into the realm of problem solving in a group dynamic.

I found that this experience—for it had passed and departed from the traditional teacher-student relationship in so grand a scale—no longer warranted the mundane title of a class. I began to confront and—sometimes—just begin to examine my own beliefs and values. I recognized that the discrepancies between seeing the world the way I do and the way the patient does had a direct impact on the care I provided and the nature and texture of the information the patient gave me. It was during this experience that I discovered the art of nursing and the benefit of therapeutic silence.

My professors—yes, they were my own private guides on this experience—were dedicated, intelligent, and motivated. I felt as though I was the only one taking the class and that the content was designed for me in particular. Learning and education had just met within me and I was now changed. Looking back on it now, I see how each interaction had its own unique purpose, leading to a common end: developing my nursing skills within the framework of what I perceived to be "me."

After graduating, to be invited to come back in the role of guide was an opportunity I could not and would not let pass me by. I have learned that in order to receive, one must learn to give freely what was given freely to *you*. I did not come to this point in my life alone, nor will I continue this journey alone. By having actual people come in and relate their experiences in class, I was afforded the opportunity to see the living, breathing part of theory.

I now look forward to the time when I am again privileged to share my life experiences with others that they too may see the flesh take hold and grow upon the skeleton of theory. I am still learning the value of giving without thought of reward, the importance of silence, and the intrinsic value of one life reaching out and perhaps touching another. I look forward to the day when I too may have the opportunity to serve as a guide.

By giving former students the opportunity to teach, we also foster continuous learning, both theirs and ours. Greg's story, and the two stories that follow, describe the importance of giving back as part of the educational process. Carrie's story describes a deep personal tragedy, one that might never have been shared if Pamela had not asked students to write about their fears as they begin the semester. Every student enters NRS 340/N341 with a wide range of "pasts" that shape the present and the future. Just as we educate students to ask questions and listen to their clients, as faculty, we should ask and listen so that we might have the opportunity to learn from our students.

CARRIE'S STORY

Carrie came into our nursing program with a prior degree. She is a bit older than some of her other classmates and clearly has a rich array of life experiences to draw on as she interacts with clients, classmates, and faculty. Carrie is bright and enthusiastic and has a good sense of humor. She is also a very mature student, who, throughout the semester in chronic illness, strove to understand and gain new meaning to a horrendous family loss. She did this by sharing her story, first in writing and later by presenting it to NRS 310 student as they were studying a unit on crisis intervention.

The Personal and Professional Challenge

What better of a way to help conquer a fear or deal with pain than to challenge it? That has been my motto for counseling myself through probably the hardest event that I have encountered in my life thus far . . . my brother's suicide. He was 21 years old.

One of the first questions I had to respond to as I began my Chronic Illness semester was, "What scares you about this clinical and what are some of the doubts, needs and resistances you'll need to overcome in order to succeed in the course?"

What a way to begin this semester. First, based on my history, I've already been dreading this particular semester of school. Now I have to reveal it all? When I saw this question on paper for the first time, I was scared to even answer it. Should I let the world know about what happened to me or should

I try to cover it up and see if I can handle it on my own without anyone's knowing my story? The answer I debated was a choice between facing my truth or hiding behind my pain. I actually contemplated the way in which I should answer this question for 2 days before actually sitting down at my computer to answer it. Finally, after contemplation and reflection, I knew what I had to do in order to grow professionally and personally. This is what I wrote:

I have a ghost in my closet, as I'm sure everyone does. I was raised in a "perfect" family of happily married parents, and one brother. My mom was a stay-at-home mom and made her career into being a great parent. Everything seemed perfect and normal until 4-and-a-half years ago.

My 21-year old brother—healthy, or so we thought—committed suicide in March of 1998. Wow!!!!!! How could a perfectly "normal" family have this happen to them? Undiagnosed depression and a well put-on act by my brother was the cause of his death.

How was I going to live with the stigma of having a family member who engaged in such a "selfish" act? That's what I would have called it prior to having this happen to me. Suddenly, this "selfish" act turned into understanding how deeply he must have hurt and how scary it was not to be able to ask for help or have anyone recognize the signs. But, I still had to live with the stigma of it all on top of my own grief.

This death postponed my return to school for several years. This is why I'm returning for my second degree at age 27 instead of 23, as originally planned. Helping my parents through this (back in Minnesota), healing my own self, and learning to live a different life is what I've been spending my last 4 years doing.

How does this clinical semester relate to my own pain and fears? I feel scared and hesitant about having to face some of what I haven't had to face yet since Ryan's death, though I'm still excited to be able to open the doors and learn a little more about people who are living with mental illness and challenges they face everyday. Will I be able to handle it? That's the question that lingers in my mind. Since I've had this personal experience, I feel much more sensitive to certain topics—especially depression and suicide—but I hope to be able to turn that anxiety into a learning experience, not only for professional growth, but even more important, for me—for my personal growth.

I'll do my best to hang in there. I may just need an extra smile once in awhile.

Well, I made it through the semester, not only feeling relieved that I was one step closer to graduation, but knowing that I had conquered one of my greatest fears: learning the basics of being a nurse for those facing both physical and mental chronic illness. I admit I did struggle a little along the way, trying not to make it apparent to anyone, but I think my own struggles helped me to feel a greater sense of accomplishment and to reap the intrinsic rewards after the fact.

Without the opportunities that we, as students, were afforded, I'm not sure that the benefit of this clinical would have been as significant for me. Almost our entire clinical time was spent this semester interacting with and learning from individuals living with chronic illness. I cannot express from the deepest part of my soul how true was the statement Pamela Minden made the first day of clinical: "You will learn as much from the residents here as they will learn from you." In my personal experience, I learned everything from them and they were my support group in challenging my pain and fear. I dedicate this part of my education to those who helped me through this experience.

I fought back the tears during my end-of-the semester conference with Pamela as I tried my hardest to express my gratitude, relief, and joy of being able to conquer this emotional semester without feeling weak or, better yet, showing my weakness. I already knew before I stepped into her office that I'd have a difficult time finding the words verbally to do this. It was the night before my conference that I decided I needed to challenge my fear one step further. I've always been a big believer in giving back to the community what you were fortunate enough to get. I stepped out of my comfort zone one more time and offered to be a guest speaker in one of the nursing classes during the next semester. Another moment of "can I really do this?" crept into my heart and soul, but I knew, deep down, that I wanted to give back.

In my previous semesters at Edgewood, we had other Edgewood alumni give of their time and share their stories during appropriate times of content in the semester. I was always touched by their personal stories and amazed by their strength, and I was able to take away and remember better the content by connecting it with the personal experiences they shared. One day, as I sat in class listening to a guest speaker and knowing that I'm always looking for more and never settling for less, I decided that, yeah, I can do this. I want to share my story, too. I want to touch lives or at least open a small window for reflection in students just starting out in their nursing education.

I feel that because this is my second time in college and I'm a little older and mom and dad aren't paying for it anymore, I've learned to take school a little more seriously. My goal as I enter any semester is to go into it open minded and ready to embrace whatever opportunities are set before me. It's all a learning experience. If I could reach out and give that mindset to all students, especially nursing students learning to deal with all of the differences in people, I certainly would. But, the next closest thing to being able to give this mindset is to try to explicitly share mine with them—from one student to another.

I had the opportunity of presenting my story during a crisis-intervention lecture to a group of 32 second-semester nursing students the following semester after my Chronic Illness Clinical semester. As I shared my personal story of my "perfect family," my college years, my brother's two college years, and then the devastating suicide, I tried to absorb the silence of the room as I watched the nursing students listening to this horrific tragedy. I was trying to deal with my own mixed emotions as I told the story, and I was hoping that they were engaged enough to listen to my true message, which was, "listen and ask." Listen to the whole person, not only concentrating on the ailment and ask the questions, even if they may make you uncomfortable. The very simplistic, yet difficult, skill of listening and expressing yourself through words is the one tool you cannot be without as a nurse. This advice is something that I've learned to be of ultimate use as I've found myself in difficult and uncomfortable situations during my journey through nursing school.

The experience one can gain from learning through a lived experience of someone else's personal life is invaluable. When you're ready to strip down to nothing and bare all that there is about yourself, you will find listeners. I'm convinced that you will touch the lives of those students who will open up their mind to listen and learn. I know that I was always one of those students trying to take in more content than possible. I needed a life situation to help me remember—something that would leave a lasting impression in my mind, something that would help me through my nursing journey.

Given this great opportunity to share my story with students, I will continue to try to reach as many open minds and eager learners as I can. And, as before, doing this convinces me that I will learn just as much from my audience as they learn from me.

We are continually surprised by the number of students who tell us, usually apologetically, that the most important learning in NRS 340 and 341 was what they learned about themselves. We delight in this revelation every time we hear it and applaud the students who share it. Providing care for others is contingent on recognizing one's own issues, strengths, and limits.

Maradee was a student who was particularly candid about how NRS 340 and 341 marked a period of great personal growth.

Maradee's Story

When we reminisce with Maradee about her time in NRS 340 and NRS 341, we recall how she always laughed at herself. Not in a disparaging way, but, rather, with sincere appreciation for how an experience humbled her. She regularly reminded us of an incident that was pivotal in her transformation from a rather cocky neophyte to a truly engaged student open to any and all learning opportunities.

Then: The Novice and the Pregnancy Test

Although we had met at clinical for a few weeks, I had not yet connected with the client, J., whom I would be interviewing. J. didn't keep to a schedule very much, and I was getting a little impatient that she kept us up. I think it was our third week at the apartment complex where J. lived when I finally met her. My classmates and instructor Pamela were having our end-of-the-day meeting when J. bounded through the door and asked, "Is Maradee here?" Since I had not met her, I wasn't sure who she was, but guessed it was J. I got up and went out in the hall to introduce myself. She was distracted and uninterested in anything that I had to say, and she interrupted me by saying, "I think I am pregnant again. I don't have any money. Will you go buy me a pregnancy test"? Out of desperate hopes of getting a real meeting with her, I said, "Sure." Some of my classmates and maybe even Pamela heard our conversation, although I am unsure. I walked back in to our meeting room and finished up for the day. The next class was gathering outside for the afternoon clinical.

I worked across the street from the apartment complex and knew that there was a pharmacy at a clinic there. After clinical, I set out for the pharmacy. That is when my common sense started to kick in. My mind was bombarded with thoughts, and I am sure I even said some of my thoughts aloud. The inappropriateness of what I was doing hit me hard.

First of all, I knew that this was no way to start off a relationship, let alone a therapeutic relationship that we had spent so much time discussing in class. I wanted J. to like me and to open up to me. I felt sorry for her because she said she had no money. I wanted to help her because she seemed so desperate and scared. I bought the test, and on the way out the door, I sat on a cold wire bench next to the entrance of the pharmacy. My heart was beating out of my chest. I was sweating. I knew what I was doing was very wrong and that I was crossing some major boundaries.

I quickly went through all the solutions to what I had done. "I just won't go back there; I can tell J. I had to work—then it will just go away and be forgotten. No, I have to go back—otherwise, she won't trust me. This is all about trust. I'll go in the back door by the dining room. That way, Pamela won't have a chance to see me. I'll tell J. not to say anything, because I shouldn't be buying things for her. I'll bring the pregnancy test over to J. after I have finished work in the evening. No, I told her I would bring it at 3 p.m. I can ask the pharmacy if they deliver." I got up and headed across the street.

I was still unsure exactly what I was going to do. I knew what I did was wrong. I didn't know Pamela, our instructor, very well, so I was sure she would lecture me and be angry if she knew what I was doing. That wouldn't be good for my clinical grade.

I made it across the street without being hit by a car, which was surprising, since I was in an altered state of mind. I walked into the apartment building through the front door and headed straight for our clinical headquarters. My thoughts were pounding in my head, "What am I doing? Just go upstairs and hand over the pregnancy test and be done with it." I raised my hand a few times to knock on the door, and by the third or fourth attempt, one of my classmates opened the door and walked out saying, "Hi, M." I don't think I answered her. Pamela saw me and invited me in. "May I talk to you?" I asked.

I sat down and Pamela pulled up a chair. I started to tell Pamela what I had done. My breath kept going away, so it was hard to speak. I sat there in fear. I knew Pamela was going to be very disappointed with me and with my actions. We talked. She asked me why I did what I did, how I felt, and why I came to her instead of taking the test to J. She could tell I wasn't my happy self. I told her my reasons. I told her all of my alternative plans of how to best get out of the situation and that I ended up here because I knew down deep it would be much better and the right thing to do to just 'fess up to what I had done. Although that sounds like the obvious choice of what to do, it was very hard for me. I wasn't the kind of person who usually did such dumb things. I usually had pretty good judgment and, after all, I had past experience working with clients like J. I knew what I was doing. I didn't need Pamela to teach me how to work with people.

Well, something clicked in me on my walk back across the street. I was going to do the right thing. I was going to grow up and take hold of my actions, right or wrong. Sitting in the chair, with Pamela across from me, I felt like a new person. I know that sounds dramatic, but I really did. I hadn't waited days to deal with what I had done, and I didn't have to hide anything or continuously justify to myself what I had done. I addressed the issue head on and really felt good.

Pamela agreed with me that what I did was wrong. I had crossed some major boundaries. She didn't berate me. She helped me talk through how I was feeling and helped me figure out how I was going to reestablish a relationship with J. that would be appropriate. After our meeting, I went to J.'s apartment, where she was eagerly waiting for me. I gave her the pregnancy test, because I had agreed to get it for her. I told her that I had to talk to her, and she agreed. I told her that it was inappropriate for her to ask me to get a pregnancy test and, most of all, that it was inappropriate for me to buy one for her. She agreed. She said that she knew I was new and that I would probably agree to it, and she took advantage of that. After that, we had a strong and appropriate student nurse/client relationship.

Pamela and I had a productive student/instructor relationship as well. I had gained great respect for Pamela and for the way she helped me instead of disciplining me. She gave me the chance to make right what I had done wrong. Most of all, Pamela allowed me to find my own inner strength, which was the greatest learning experience of all.

During the semester that she was in the chronic illness courses, Maradee also completed an independent study focused on end-of-life care. She trained with the local hospice organization and became a valued volunteer. Not only did she provide services for dying clients and their families, she also assisted in training other volunteers. To document her learning, she developed a PowerPoint presentation that included photographs she took in a required Edgewood art class that showed her reflections on the meaning of service. We were so impressed by the quality of this work that we asked her to teach the academic class period devoted to end-of-life concerns. She describes what it meant for her to evolve from student to teacher.

Now: The Hospice Expert

I was invited to present my independent project to my graduating class instead of the normal meeting with the Human Issues coordinators for completion of my project. This is how I became a student who was teaching a class on death and dying at Edgewood College. To better understand my experience, it may be helpful to have some background information.

Edgewood has a requirement that all students fulfill a Human Issues project requirement prior to graduation. This can be completed in a number of ways, one of which is to have a volunteer experience. I didn't want to have to commit to a class and was looking forward to a new volunteer experience. I had always volunteered to do things that were fun and comfortable—things like literacy tutoring, yard work for shut-ins, and special events at the nursing home. I was trying to think of something fun to do. I was talking to my mum on the phone, and she suggested I try something out of my comfort range. For all of my life, my mother has encouraged me to try different things, things out of my comfort zone. My uncle Dave had been a hospice volunteer, and, for some reason, I grabbed onto that idea. I had worked with dying people for many years, and some friends and family members have died. Outwardly, I handled death OK. Inwardly, it freaked me out.

After getting approval for my Human Issues project, arranging it with the local Hospice and completing their extensive hospice training program and volunteering at the inpatient part of the hospice center, I agreed to my first in-home volunteer assignment. Three months later, after my first client passed away, I took on a second in-home assignment. A month later, my second client passed away. For the sake of brevity, I'm not going to talk about my experience as a hospice volunteer directly. Instead, I'm going to write about my experience of presenting my volunteer experience to my classmates, instructors, and other nursing students.

When discussing how I would package my final presentation to the Human Issues department, I thought it would be fun to put together a PowerPoint presentation rather than writing yet another paper. I received permission from both my Human Issues advisor, Pamela, and from the point person in the Human Issues department. I started working on my presentation right away because I just wanted to be done with this requirement. As I was building my presentation, I thought of using some black-and-white photographs I had taken in my required art class at Edgewood. After a lot of work, I had more than the average PowerPoint presentation. I admit I was very proud of what I had created. My plan was to show the presentation to Pamela and Malathi, my Human Issues point person, and be done with it. Pamela asked to see my work, and after she viewed my presentation, she asked if I would show it to my class and discuss my experience with them, since our death and dying content was coming up. Immediately, and without thinking, I said no. That was way too intimidating for me. I was sure that they wouldn't understand how important and life changing this volunteer experience had been to me. I didn't want to share with them this soft part of me. I was a member of this class, and I knew that they wouldn't be interested in what I had to show them or say to them. Yes, they would be polite because it was me, but they wouldn't "get it."

After a week or so and after more editing of my presentation, Pamela asked me if I would reconsider presenting to my class. I gave in. I figured if she wanted me to so badly, I would and could. I would also invite Malathi so that I wouldn't have to present twice. Building up to the day of my presentation, I was constantly trying to make my presentation better. I added pictures, changed fonts and layouts, wrote my comments so I would remember what to say, and made four copies on various media so that I would be sure that the presentation would technically work.

The night before my presentation, I planned what clothes I would wear, and edited my creation once again. The next morning I arrived early to make sure the equipment was ready and working. I was beyond nervous. Pamela introduced me as she would any guest speaker. I thought, "What is she doing? They know who I am." I prefaced my presentation with a bit of background information and then turned out the lights. I started my presentation. It was deadly silent. Later I heard sniffling. It was the cold season, I thought. I came to the end, and the lights in the room went on. My classmates were looking at me in a daze, some with red, glassy eyes, some still sniffling, and one just letting the tears roll down her cheeks. Pamela and Malathi just stared at me. Then they all clapped. Honestly, I had no idea what to do. I thought they were just moved because, near the end, I quoted my last interaction with the last lady whom I had volunteered with. It was a moving quote. Pamela suggested we take a break, and when everyone came back, we would talk about my presentation. Good idea.

My classmates told me what a visually pleasing PowerPoint presentation I had made. They told me, "Good job," and then they started asking questions: How did I feel knowing these people were going to die? How did I feel when they died? How did I ever decide to volunteer at hospice? One of my classmates said, "This experience really changed you, didn't it, M.?" It had, and with her invitation to talk about it, I did talk about it a little bit. I talked about how not only had this experience deeply affected my sense of self, but it also taught me a lot about how I interact with those around me. I gained a deep sense of self-awareness from this experience. My classmates accepted me as a guest speaker. I wasn't just M, standing up and talking. I was talking about something important to me. What I had not expected was that what I was talking about would be important to them.

After my successful completion of my Human Issues project presentation, I thought I was done with it. A few weeks after my original presentation, Pamela asked me if I would present my experience to the class next semester when they would be on the topic of death and dying. I agreed. I had gained unexpected acceptance from my own class—presenting to a class that was not full of my peers would be no problem.

Well, the next semester came. I showed up early in the morning and did my presentation. The lights came on, and the class looked at me blankly. Silence. No comments. Blank expressions. One student was sleeping. They didn't get it. Initially, I was ready to pack up and leave. They could do what they wanted with what I just shared with them. Then one student raised her hand and asked me, "Wasn't it hard to take another patient after your first one died?" That was a start. I talked to them about the fears I had and the feelings I experienced. Another student asked me why I chose this project. Another asked if the patients even wanted me there. There were lots of good questions. Thankfully, this class got some value out of what I had taught them. I was afraid that they wouldn't.

Returning to be a guest speaker/expert in a program in which I was still a student was initially very difficult for me. Like my hospice volunteer experience, it was out of my comfort zone. I also found it hard to believe that Pamela really thought I was an expert at something, let alone a topic that *she* was supposed to be teaching. I was honored that she and other instructors were interested in what I had to say. I learned that we all had a lot to learn from each other. I was now in a new peer group of teachers. It was surprising to me when other instructors stopped me in the hall to ask if they could come to my next presentation. I decided to embrace my feeling of being proud of what I had done.

As for dealing with the extreme reactions of those students whom I presented to, it took me a while to figure out what to do. Initially, I felt that since this experience had been so great for me, it must also be great for them. I learned quickly that that was not the case, and being a guest presenter would be more and more difficult if that was my expectation. I learned to go with the flow. I later prefaced my presentation with the thought that we are all in very different places in our lives, and we are all affected differently by what we experience. "Of course, I hope you find at least one thing from my experience that gives you something to think about, but if you don't, that is OK, too." I tell the students that this project started out with my desire to fulfill my Human Issues requirement early, but, instead, it changed my life. Some students got that, others didn't. If nothing else, I think that my presentation helps students consider how they feel about death. They may not verbalize it, but I bet they think about it. If they get more than that from my presentation, that is great.

What I have come to realize is that being a guest presenter has taught me more about myself than how to be a good teacher. Yes, I am there to teach, but I hope that those who hear my story, learn that it isn't always about *what* you are doing but what you are *learning* by doing it. I end my presentation by giving the same advice to my "students" as my mother continues to give to me. "Try something that is out of your comfort zone. It can be something tiny or something huge, but just try. You may be amazed by your own strength."

CONCLUSION

Successful completion of class assignments and exams is one indication that most of our students have mastered the content necessary to progress in the nursing program, and, ultimately, to succeed on the licensure exam. Becoming and being an accomplished nurse requires so much more, though. The Edgewood Nursing Department, as indicated in its vision statement, seeks to develop competent nurses who are passionate about their profession, who are committed to life-long learning, and who are dedicated to the promotion of holistic health, peace, and justice. This is a tall order—and it is an order in which success is difficult to measure. At the beginning of each semester, we set out to achieve the prespecified objectives for each course, but the truth is, we never know exactly where the students, or we, will end up. Many students tell us that they learned a lot in the chronic illness courses, though not all can articulate the specifics and wholeness of what that was as clearly as Greg, Carrie, and Maradee.

Another piece of feedback we often receive from our students, which gratifies us to no end, is that they learn in the chronic illness courses to see, be, and think differently. James P. Carse notes that we know we have met a master teacher "when we come away amazed not at what the teacher was thinking but at what we were thinking" (1994, p. 70). We aspire to be that sort of teacher, inspiring our students to recognize and use their own unique gifts.

The chronic illness courses are situated smack in the middle of a nursing program that fits within a larger context of a liberal arts education. Though it is impossible for us to isolate what specifically we have added to the scholarly development of any one of our students, we know that this pair of courses makes some difference in how students conceive of chronic illness and in their ability to respond to people living a life with it. Their written and oral stories, some of which are conveyed in chapters 4 and 5 (and also above), reveal new recognition that people are more than the labels applied to them, and a greater openness to working with a population many had previously ruled out because they perceived chronic care as boring and filled with hopelessness. We close this chapter and book with one last story—a small but nonetheless poignant illustration of such transformation.

Because Maradee Said So

In planning for the wellness group required in the psychosocial-spiritual component of the clinical course, one cohort of students who succeeded Maradee's graduating class decided to illustrate the mind-body connection by providing the clients with foot baths and massages. They hypothesized that such a nurturing experience would promote both mental and physical ease. That is, all but one did. "I draw the line at touching feet! I will help in some other way, but I refuse to wash or fondle anybody's dirty feet." Though she was willing to do whatever else the session leader would require of her, Sharon was adamant that she could not bear to smell, much less come into physical contact with, another's feet. Though she could not counter her peers' admonishment that she would at some point in her nursing career have to face up to this fear, she would not budge.

The students went ahead with their plans but agreed to accommodate Sharon by allowing her to provide hand massages instead. The foot session happened to follow the week of Maradee's hospice presentation in NRS 340. On the day of the event, Pamela was quite surprised to find Sharon spontaneously genuflect in front of an obese, rather disheveled man and gently take off his shoes and socks. Astonishingly, her confident and comfortable demeanor belied the distress she had in prior weeks said she experienced just in thinking about doing such a thing. Even more amazingly, once she lovingly patted dry his feet and restored his shoes and socks to their rightful spot, she moved on to repeat the task with several other clients.

By the time the session ended and the debriefing began, Pamela was nearly bursting at the seams to inquire about Sharon's behavior but forced herself to follow the usual protocol.

What was the experience like for the leader? Would she like feedback, and if so, what kind? What did the students learn in the session that could enhance their ability to provide care for people living a life with chronic illness? Finally, unable to restrain herself further Pamela blurted, "Sharon, you *knocked my socks off* when you took off Joe's shoes and socks! I couldn't believe my eyes! What happened?"

Sharon simply smiled demurely and replied, "I just kept thinking about Maradee saying how important it is to do things outside your comfort zone."

REFERENCES

Carse, J. P. (1995). *Breakfast at the victory: The mysticism of ordinary experience.* San Francisco: Harper Collins.

Palmer, P. (1998). *The courage to teach.* San Francisco: Jossey-Bass.

Case Examples

olleen has written up a number of stories from her clinical practice and personal experience illustrating key scientific principles and providing an opening into discussion of the various ways a nurse might intervene, depending on how the scenario unfolds. These narratives provide students with an opportunity to integrate *living a life* with theoretical knowledge in such a way that blending the art and science of nursing practice is enabled. The first case study demonstrates how content related to COPD and emphysema can be designed to emphasize pulmonary rehabilitation principles. The academic content that can be interwoven with the case studies are printed in **bold** type.

Uncle Lee (Emphysema)

In the fall of my sophomore year in nursing school, my father's oldest brother, Uncle Lee, died from emphysema. At the time, I really didn't know anything about emphysema except that Uncle Lee had been getting worse and worse in the last 10 years, and now he was dead. At that time, 10 years seemed like a very long time to be ill.

What can I say about my Uncle Lee? He was a really neat guy with a very dry sense of humor. I remember watching him interact with his wife, Aunt Stella. It was sort of like watching George Burns and Gracie Allen. But the neatest thing I remember about Uncle Lee was that he rolled his own cigarettes, lots of them. My brother and I would sit on the living room floor and watch him in amazement as he methodically rolled one cigarette after another. I remember when he was first diagnosed with emphysema. Everyone said it was because he had worked in the iron mines up in Minnesota as a boy. No one ever suspected cigarettes.

Types of Lung Diseases
  Restrictive
  Obstructive
  Emphysema
  Chronic Bronchitis

Our family would visit my aunt and uncle often. Either we would go to their house or they would come over to ours. Uncle Lee drove a maroon Buick and always wore white starched shirts. As his disease progressed, their visits became less frequent. I remember how difficult it was for him to walk into the house from the car. He would have to stop two or three times just to catch his breath. Even this small amount of exercise would send him into a coughing fit that would last for several minutes. Aunt Stella would get really mad at him for coughing so much. Once in the house, he always sat on the very edge of the sofa, always leaning forward. His shoulders were always up as high as he could get them, like someone permanently shrugging their shoulders. Uncle Lee said there was a pulmonary specialist in Milwaukee who wanted to treat him. He had enrolled in a pulmonary rehab. program at St. Mary's hospital. Aunt Stella wasn't very optimistic, nor was she very supportive, "I don't know what he wants to go way down there for, anyway," she'd grumble.

Fundamentals of Pulmonary Rehabilitation
Smoking Cessation (the most important change)
Methods:
  Patient and family education
  Exercise training
  Goals:
  Methods:
    Oxygen therapy
    Criteria for use:
    Oxygen dose

As the years progressed, Uncle Lee got worse and worse. He became very thin. His pants hung on him like a child wearing his father's clothes. He didn't smoke anymore—not because he didn't want to, I'm sure, but because he was simply too short of breath. He was on home oxygen now. I really never know much about what medications he was taking, but every once in a while, I remember seeing him pull out an inhaler. It looked very difficult to use because he could barely take in a deep breath. He would often sit and listen to the rest of us talk and occasionally provide an affirmative nod to let us know that, even though he couldn't physically participate in the conversation, he was still following us.

Medical Management:
  Vaccinations
  Corticosteroids
  Bronchodilators
  Antibiotics
  Surgery
  Lung Reduction

Additional Nursing Issues:
Rest and sleep
Nutrition

My parents called me one night in October to say Uncle Lee had died at St. Mary's hospital. He was 68. The doctor had talked with Aunt Stella and their son Milton about whether or not to intubate him. The decision was made against intubation. Uncle Lee was buried on a beautiful, sunny, crisp October day. Three years later, the reality of Uncle Lee's death hit home to my father, who likewise was developing emphysema. My dad was a very heavy smoker—4 packs per day. He decided one day to quit. In his own words, "enough is enough." It wasn't easy for him. For about 24 hours afterwards, he became physically ill with nicotine withdrawal, experiencing nausea, vomiting, and diarrhea. He knew what it was, but as he looked back on it, he would laughingly say, "the sicker I got, the more I knew I would never smoke again." I'm glad he made that decision—too bad it wasn't soon enough. My dad died of lung cancer 20 years after he quit smoking.

Another example of shifting content to focus on tertiary prevention can be seen in the class session dedicated to nursing management of diabetes. Information related to chronic complications is presented first, followed by daily management issues such as glycemic control and medication management. Last, information addressing the management of hypoglycemia is discussed. Management of acute diabetic ketoacidosis or hyperglycemic coma is addressed in a subsequent course.

Dickey: Everybody Needs a Nurse (Diabetes)

My husband, Rick, owns a small trucking company. This was how we met Dickey. Dickey drove a truck for my husband for about 2 years. It was the summer of 1988, the second hottest summer on record, when Dickey started working for Rick. Dickey was a huge Swedish fellow, about 6-feet-5 inches tall and weighing 250 pounds. He previously worked as a cheese maker in Monroe. I heard he was very good at it, but he got tired of making cheese and decided to become a truck driver instead. Dickey made it no secret that he had diabetes; in fact, he was quite at ease about having insulin vials and syringes in the refrigerator down at the shop. Rick said everyday Dickey carried insulin syringes and orange juice in his lunch box. Once in a while, though, he would comment to Rick about how the doctors had been warning him about how "loose" he was in controlling his blood sugar levels. Dickey just laughed. I don't know how long he had been diagnosed with diabetes, but in 1988, Dickey was only 44 years old.

Who Gets Diabetes?
Diagnosing diabetes

Blood values
Types of Diabetes (Type 1 and Type 2)

After 2 years of driving for Rick, Dickey decided to buy his own truck and lease it out for work. He drove an old White Constructor. By this time, it was no secret to anyone remotely connected to trucking that Dickey liked his beer. His favorite was Huber beer out of Monroe. In fact, Dickey had a huge sign on the front grill of his truck that said HUBER. Everyone called him Huber. Once in a while he'd stop in to see Rick. During one visit he said he had been in the hospital twice that summer to "jump start" his heart. He said the doctors told him he really needed to start watching his diabetes more closely because there would come a time when they couldn't keep shocking his heart. This bothered Dickey, and after every hospitalization, he would do better in managing his diabetes. After a few months, though, everything was back to "normal." Besides, who has time for this illness anyway? Dickey was known as a fun-loving kind of guy.

Chronic Complications (Who gets them?)
General patient education about chronic complications
Vascular Complications: large (macrovascular) & small (microvascular) vessel disease
Atherosclerosis
Hyperlipidemia
Kidney: nephropathy
Retina: retinopathy—proliferative and nonproliferative diabetic retinopathy

As years went by, we would hear from Dickey and his wife Mary Kay a couple of times a year. They had two children: an 11-year-old boy nicknamed Duke (as in John Wayne) and a 6-year-old girl named Deanna. Last December the family stopped by for a visit. Dickey was thinking of buying a different truck. Mary Kay had acquired the responsibility of truck mechanic and would do the greasing, oil changes, tire changes, and so on. Duke was into horses. The family owned two or three, and Duke would go with his friends to ride horseback every day after school. Deanna and our daughter, Heather, immediately hit it off playing Barbies. At that time, Dickey talked to us about his health and how he was having trouble with his feet. He said they always felt like they were asleep and were always cold.

Neuropathies (distal symmetrical polyneuropathy, visceral-autonomic)
Orthostatic hypotension
GI
GU
Sexuality

Early this summer, we heard that Dickey was in the hospital. We heard rumors that he had his leg cut off. Then we heard he had both legs cut off, then we heard he had part of a foot cut off. In August, Rick stopped by Dickey's house to see how he was doing. It's been 14 years since we first met Dickey. He is now 54. Dickey said it all started with a new pair of steel-tip work shoes that didn't fit quite right. They rubbed his foot the wrong way and gave him blisters. One thing led to another. The local doctors were trying to treat them, and they prescribed whirlpool treatments two or three times a week. At this particular hospital, a vascular specialist comes out once a week. When he first saw Dickey's foot, he drained pus out of his blisters and told Dickey he had gangrene, that his foot would have to come off *right now*. Dickey told Rick that same day they took him to the university hospital and did the amputation. He had part of his foot taken off, but after surgery, he ended up back in the hospital two more times because of delayed healing and post-op infections.

FOOT CARE, FOOT CARE, FOOT CARE, FOOT CARE ! ! !
Risk factors
Examining feet (What are you looking for?)
Nursing assessments/teaching

That visit was particularly hard for my husband, Rick. He came home and talked about it for a long time. It was about 11:00 a.m. when he went to visit. Rick said Dickey was still in bed. Mary Kay was at work, and the two kids were supposedly in charge of taking care of dad and the household. He said Dickey had lost a lot of weight—four pants sizes Dickey told him. He also told Rick he could hardly see out of his left eye anymore and that his left arm was starting to get weak. There was a wheelchair sitting next to the bed. Dickey said his leg hurt so badly when it was in a dependent position that he hardly got out of bed anymore. He tried a car ride once, but Dickey said, "What's the sense of going for a car ride when you have to lie down in the back of the car? You can't see anything anyway." The picture of the small, cramped house, the two young kids at home, and Dickey in bed left a vivid memory in Rick's mind. All he could say when he got home was, "How did all this happen, how did he get so bad?" After thinking about it even longer, Rick said, "He's never going to be able to work again, will he?" I said probably not and that Dickey would most likely end up on disability—if he's lucky.

Tertiary Care
Monitoring glycemic control
Who should use what type?
Urine testing
Capillary blood glucose monitoring (CBG)
Glycosylated hemoglobin (HgbA1C)

I'd like to think that Dickey wouldn't be where he is today if he had a really good diabetic nurse working with him. Strategies for managing diabetes are pretty clear cut, the trick is integrating them into the life of a beer drinking wild and crazy truck-driver kind of guy. We health care providers can provide information until the cows come home. The really good health care providers help people like Dickey figure out what to do with the information and how to live a life with diabetes.

Art of Diabetes Management

Talking with folks about changing lifelong habits is, at best, a very difficult topic. Habits, such as how we eat and what we do with the little spare time we have, are changed by choice, not information. Clients like Dickey are challenging, but the secret is to start slowly and gradually integrate changes.

Daily Management
Diet:
  General goals
  Target weight
  Carbohydrates
  Proteins
  Fats
Special considerations for Type 2 clients
Special considerations for Type 1 clients

People's concepts of what constitutes exercise in interesting and entertaining. If you ever want to get a rise out of someone, try telling a farmer that the work he or she does isn't exercise. Everyone thinks they exercise. You might get further by acknowledging their level of activity and hard work but then talk about a different type of exercise program.

Exercise
  Aerobic activity
  Benefits
  Assessment before starting
Exercise prescription
  Program objectives
  Types of exercise
  Adjustments in food intake or insulin

As if diet, exercise, and monitoring blood sugars weren't enough to be bothered with in managing diabetes, then add the extra confusion of insulin management.

Medications
  Insulins
    Time-action curves
    Mixtures

Dosage Adjustments
Mixing insulins
Storage
Things to consider re: SQ injection of insulin and site selection
Oral antidiabetic agents

Try and imagine an individual or family like Dickey's that is struggling to manage the complexities of this illness. It takes time. It would be wonderful if all our clients were perfect and checked their blood sugars four times a day, followed their diets, exercised, and took their insulin correctly, but this just isn't all that common. In fact, there are probably a lot of Dickeys out in the world. As if this weren't enough information, there is one more piece of information that all folks taking medications for glycemic control *must* know:

Signs and symptoms of *hypoglycemia*
  Adrenergic symptoms
  Cholinergic symptoms
  Neuroglycopenic symptoms

Glenn: What Medicine Can't Do (Hypertension)

I've heard it said that when you marry a man, you marry his family. I guess that's true for me. Glenn and Gladys, Rick's parents, best epitomized the challenges health care providers face when providing care to folks with un-usual health beliefs, few financial resources, and limited education. Glenn had stage 3 hypertension and many of the long-term effects of target organ disease (TOD). Gladys is totally healthy. Glenn relied on prescription drugs (a lot of them) to control his blood pressure; Gladys relied on her own concoction of herbs, creams—and, most important, her staple—vinegar and honey. She attributed her good health to her home remedies and Glenn's continued hypertension and poor health on unknowledgeable doctors and nurses, "They don't know what they're doing." Glenn always carried a card in his wallet with his blood pressure (BP) readings. He'd pull it out from time to time and show me—like a service record for your car with the oil changes. It was as if this card insured him for good health. He could look at all those readings and somehow pretend his hypertension wasn't as bad as it really was.

Diagnosing hypertension
Risk Factors:

1. **Smoking**
2. **Elevated lipids (dyslipidemia)**
3. **Diabetes**

4. Age
5. Gender
6. Family History

Stages of Hypertension
Health Beliefs

Glenn had his first myocardial infarction (MI) at age 54. This was around 1980. Of course, he denied it, "Just some indigestion. Those doctors don't know what they're doing, all they want is my money." By the 1990s he was having transient ischemic attacks (TIAs). One day, he was driving a school bus and started having TIA symptoms. Thank God he had dropped off his last kid and was driving an empty bus. We begged the Dr. to help Glenn retire from driving. It finally happened. Activities were difficult for Glenn. We would just shake our heads, as he would start up the bus just to drive 10 feet to get the mail. His home had lots of stairs. No wonder he would plan his day to only have to go up and down once or twice a day. It was not uncommon for him to have to take 5–6 nitro tablets just to get up one flight of stairs.

Target Organ Disease:
  Cardiovascular:
  Neurological:
  Renal disease:
  Vascular disease:
  Retinopathy:
Lifestyle Changes:
  Diet:
  Exercise:
  Weight reduction
  Alcohol:
  Smoking:
  Stress Management:

By now, Glenn's medical regimen had become quite complex and expensive. Of course, he had very little health insurance. I'm sure he'd pick and choose which drugs he'd take. Gladys always supplemented Glenn's meds with garlic, vinegar, honey, and whatever else she'd heard about at the beauty parlor. When he'd start having chest pain, instead of his prn NTG, she'd rub his shoulders with the massager. He was supposed to wear NTG patches at all times to prevent angina. Glenn felt that if he wasn't having pain, why should he waste the patches. After all, they cost 50 cents apiece. It made more sense to him to wait until he had chest pain to use the medication than to try and prevent attacks.

Medication Management

It wasn't uncommon for Glenn to be hospitalized 2–3 times each year for complications from HTN. We'd get these emergency calls at any time, day or night . . . "Would you come over? Glenn's having trouble." It got to be the family joke. Rick got to know all the ED personnel and folks in admission at our local hospital. He knew the routine—be sure to take Glenn's wallet; it had all his health cards in it. His doctor said he had one severe stenosis in one area of his heart that was causing the problems. He had completely occluded his RCA with his first MI.

October 23, 1996. It was 2:30 a.m. Gladys called again. "Please come over. Glenn is really bad." I remember cursing in the closet as I threw on some clothes. "If he'd just take his meds like he's supposed to, we wouldn't have this trouble all the time." I was really upset. When I got there, I knew right away that this would be Glenn's last trip to the ED. Clearly, he was in pulmonary edema. I thought to myself, "He must have finally infarcted that last part of his heart." I called Rick and told him to get over here, this was it. We called 911. They responded quickly. As they loaded Glenn into the ambulance in the driveway, I heard him breathe his last breath. He was dead when he arrived at the hospital.

Candy and Sally: Arthritis Isn't Just for Old People

I've only known two people in my lifetime with rheumatoid arthritis (RA). Their stories probably best represent the extremes of the disease. They were both young women.

I first met Sally when I was an advisor for a senior-high youth group. I was a recent graduate nurse and knew absolutely nothing about arthritis. Why should I? Only old people get arthritis, right? Not quite. Sally was only 16 when I met her. I didn't know she had arthritis when I first met her. It's not exactly one of those diseases you can always detect. The more I interacted with her, though, the more I began to put things together. Then, one day, we were sitting around playing cards. She was awful at shuffling. Everyone kept on saying, "Come on Sally. What's taking you so long? Just pass out the cards." While she fumbled around with the cards, I caught a glance of her hands and fingers. It wasn't hard to miss. At the age of 16, she had already undergone extensive surgical procedure to replace joints. The tops of her hands were covered with scars.

What is arthritis?
Types of arthritis
  RA:
  OA (DJD)
  Gout

Candy, on the other hand, was the extreme opposite of Sally. Candy was a fellow undergraduate nursing student. She was by far one of the funniest people I have ever met. Her rendition of her first injection had us all rolling on the floor laughing. She was thin and very active. She ran in 10k races before running was even popular. She never missed a day of school. She never told many people about her arthritis. I just happened to overhear one of her conversations one day with a nursing instructor explaining why she was late for clinical. Of course, that did help explain the jumbo size bottle of ASA she carried around. No one has that many headaches, not even a nursing student.

Diagnosing Arthritis
  Pain and joint stiffness:
    RA
    OA
  Joints involved:
    RA
    OA
  Other systemic issues:

One year, our senior-high group was planning on doing volunteer work down south in Arkansas. Sally was planning on going but had concerns about the long car ride, sleeping on the floors of church basements in sleeping bags, and the nature of the work we would be doing (painting houses, washing windows, doing yard work, digging trenches, and so forth). Not exactly the type of work someone with arthritis would normally be doing. You could tell by the way she walked she was never very comfortable.

Sally really had some hard years as a teen. Her parents were quite wealthy. She had one younger brother. It was difficult balancing dependence with independence. When Sally would need to rest her joints, people thought she was slacking. When others would help her by carrying her books, people said they were playing to Sally's obsession with her illness. Others said she was manipulative and used her disease to get what she wanted. Some friends were overprotective and offered too much help; others offered no help at all. It was a continuous balancing act. Sally was very bright at school and wanted to study to be an architect.

Management Issues
  Goals of Management
  Methods of pain control:
    Positioning
    Splinting
    Thermal modalities
    Rest
    Exercise
    Joint protection

Relaxation techniques
Transcutaneous electrical nerve stimulation
Pharmacological management
  Pain control and disease modifying
  OA: (know drugs, maximum dose, and side effect)
    First line:
    Second line:
  RA: First-line drugs
    Second-line drugs

Candy, on the other hand, continued to do well as a student. About 3 years after graduation, I moved back to Milwaukee, and by coincidence ended up working in the same intensive care unit (ICU) as Candy. I remember sitting in report one day and hearing this familiar laugh, and, much to my surprise, it was Candy. She still was active but had changed her sport from running to swimming. She said she had good days and bad days but, overall, most of her days were pretty good. She did say that 12 hour shifts were pretty difficult for her. She was thinking about starting a family and was concerned about how she would manage her meds if she got pregnant.

Living with Arthritis:
  Joint protection:
    Splinting
      Decrease or eliminate pain
      Decrease inflammation
      Decrease symptoms of nerve entrapment
      Support ligament and joint capsules
      Correct or minimize deformities/contractures
      Stabilize for function
    Exercise
      Do on good days and bad days
      Decrease repetitions during severe inflammation
      Respect pain
      Use active exercises whenever possible
      Do not substitute ADLs for exercises
      Avoid resistance during severe inflammation
    Ambulation devices
      Increases safety
      Decreases stress on lower extremities
      Reduces pain in weight bearing joints
      Compensates for unstable or weak joints
      Increases independence
    Assistive devices
      Maintain and/or increase independence
      Simplify tasks

Reduce pain in accomplishing tasks
Minimize extraneous stress on joints
Joint replacement

It has been almost a decade since I have seen either Candy or Sally. Since writing this, I really wonder what has become of either of them. I'm sure Candy is doing well and probably has several children by now. I'm not so sure about Sally. She was already receiving gold injections as a teen.

I have since grown to understand how incapacitating RA can be. It's not just a disease of the joints—it can rob a person of his or her energy as well. Depression among those with RA is quite common. Today, new drugs are being developed that help prevent the extensive joint destruction so common with RA, but these drugs are expensive and are not tolerated by everyone. I can't help but wonder if Candy's children will develop her disease as well.

Sample Wellness Interviews

SAMPLE 1

Name of Interviewer: Student 1   Date: 9/25/03

Client Wellness Interview Summary

Client Description

Client Initials: B.W.   Gender: Male
Age: 48   Marital Status: separated, in a 3-
                                          year relationship with girlfriend

Client Perspective on Wellness

How does the client describe wellness?
B.W. describes wellness as being able to maintain a daily routine. Being able to get up, get yourself fed, and entertain yourself. Just functioning on a daily basis.

Does the client regard himself or herself as well?
Wouldn't describe himself as well. Has many physical ailments. Is overweight and suffers with COPD and back pain related to his injury.

Can the client articulate any wellness goals?
Has lost some weight but would really like to lose some additional weight. Wants to quit smoking because he has problems with breathing.

Spirit. (Use spiritual assessment tools as appropriate—available on blackboard)

Spiritual orientation, traditions, customs
B.W. believes in God and believes that there is a meaning for him being here on earth, but has not yet figured out what that meaning is. Has faith in God and explained that when he was in his accident at work, it wasn't his time to go. Has thought about death and what happens after death but is still uncertain as to what he thinks will happen after we die. Does believe that life continues after death, but doesn't necessarily believe in a heaven or hell.

Religious affiliation
He did not mention what type of faith he believes in besides God in general and that he does not preach about religion or go to church. Said that spirituality really does not play a part in his life right now.

Values and beliefs

1. *What is important in your life?* Currently, B.W is focused on getting the lawsuit regarding his work injury settled. This issue is very stressful to him because he has past due bills and needs to be able to put this behind him.
2. *What gives your life meaning?* It seems that B.W. is future oriented and has certain goals that he is looking forward to meeting. Relationship with D. is very important and he has hopes to move into a house with her. Is also in contact with his children by phone every week.

Mind. Mental Status Assessment: *Discerned through observation and questioning. Feel free to experiment with any screening tools you'd like and be sure to include any abnormal findings.*

General Description (appearance, motor activity, speech pattern, general attitude): B.W. was dressed in a T-shirt and sweat pants and wore a baseball cap. His shirt was slightly dirty and he was wearing a lot of cologne. Uses his hands to gesture while he speaks—appropriate movements.

Emotions (mood and affect): B.W. said he is normally in a good mood and was in an okay mood the day of our interview. He was very pleasant, respective and cooperative. Throughout the interview, he maintained good eye contact.

Thought Process (observe rate & flow of speech, associations made, logical flow)

1. *Form.* His speech was clear and flowed logically. He spoke in an appropriate tone and manner for our discussion and environment.

2. *Content.* Very logical and pertaining to our conversation. Thoughts are well organized and flow well. Answers promptly, but sometimes pauses as if he is organizing his thoughts before answering. Will ask for clarification if he does not understand my questions. His thoughts are well associated; he does not get distracted and sticks to the topics being discussed.

Perception: Client makes sense. Appears to be consistently aware of reality.

Sensorium and Cognition

1. *Orientation.* Alert and orientated to person, place, time, and circumstances.
2. *Memory.* Suffers from some short-term memory problems related to head injury.
3. *Calculation.* Did not assess in depth. Able to perform simple calculations, demonstrated by ability to subtract a number of years since his accident or since he began dating D. and then, also, giving the answer pertaining to the year of the accident and when he started dating D.

Impulse Control. Did not assess. Does not seem like he is impulsive or at risk for impulsive behavior.

Judgment and Insight

1. *Ability to solve problems.* Client has been successful in the past with solving problems he has faced up to this point in his life. He knows when he needs help and will ask his girlfriend or Kate for assistance or reminders when it comes to his memory loss. Is capable of abstract thinking. Able to be of assistance to others (e.g., to girlfriend) when they are in need of help.
2. *Ability to make decisions.* Client is independent and capable of making the decisions needed to take care of himself and to control his situation and environment. Knows when he needs to ask others for help.
3. *Knowledge about self.* Knows what areas he needs to improve in, such as losing weight and quitting smoking. Doesn't always give himself credit for his good qualities and his ability to help and care for others in their time of need.

4. *Coping and/or defense mechanisms.* B.W. seems to cope with problems as they come up by talking issues through with his girlfriend
and Kate. As for defense mechanisms, B.W. may use suppression
as a way to live with not seeing his children. He said he has just
learned to live without them and maybe he tries blocking his
feelings regarding this issue.

Body. Check any of *Roy's physiological modes* in which there are concerns
or needs. Comment on what they are.

Mode	Comments
Activity & rest: (ambulation, ADL, sleep, energy level)	Performs some exercises and stretches to loosen up his back. Does stomach crunches while in bed. Cannot walk long distances without using his oxygen tank. Would like to do low impact exercises to get his heart rate up and burn calories.
Nutrition (height, weight, diet)	Tries to eat healthily by eating vegetables. Gained a lot of weight after his accident but has recently lost some of the weight—Is trying to lose more
Elimination (problems, concerns, recent changes)	Not directly assessed
Oxygenation (smoker?)	Currently is smoking. Wants to quit, as he has difficulties with breathing. Suffers from COPD as well. Sleeps with oxygen on, but doesn't use it when walking short distances because he says it is a hassle
Fluid and electrolytes	Not directly assessed
Endocrine	Not directly assessed
Protection (any fall risk?)	Due to his back pain and previously broken pelvis, he would be unable to get up off of the floor if he did fall. Uses a van for

	transportation as it is easier to get into and out of for him
Senses (sight, hearing, pain)	Always in pain related to (R/T) his back and pelvis
Neurological	Head injury R/T accident at work. Suffered from depression after his accident. Not currently suffering from or taking anything for depression. Now has some short term memory problems
Reproductive (sexuality)	Implied he is sexually active with girlfriend. Does not want more children, already has three. Had past problems with priapism R/T Zoloft for depression

Medication Profile

List *all* medications (PRNs included) client currently takes.	Uses aspirin. Takes oxycontin and oxycodone for pain management. Used to take Tylenol and damaged his liver. Now is very careful of taking medications that can harm the liver or anything with Tylenol in it. Previously was taking Zoloft for depression.

Milieu. Psychosocial & Environmental Concerns: DSM IV–Axis IV (Indicate strengths & deficits)

Mode	Comments
1. Primary support group	Primarily his girlfriend. Still close to some of his family. Has some acquaintances at the Triangle Community Ministry Parish (the "Triangle"), but not many close friends he would share his problems with. Counts on his girlfriend and Kate for most of his support

2. Social environment	Lives at the Triangle with his girl-friend. Doesn't have many close friends at the Triangle—does have people he considers to be acquaintances. He has three children who he still keeps in touch with over the phone. Has learned to accept that he cannot see them and only talks to them
3. Education	Not assessed
4. Occupation	Not currently employed. Due to his accident, he had work restrictions in place and it was too hard on his back
5. Housing	Currently living at the Triangle since 2000. Hopes to someday live in a house with his girlfriend
6. Economics	Low income. Has past due bills R/T accident and workman's compensation running out. Needs the lawsuit to be settled so he can pay bills
7. Access to health care services	Returns to the rehab unit at UW once a month. Sees a Rehab specialist there
8. Interaction with the legal system	Lawsuit regarding the fall at work
9. Other—specify	N/A

Nursing Diagnosis: List nursing diagnoses for any problems or needs that were apparent:

1. Activity intolerance R/T COPD and back pain manifested by (M/B) inability to walk long distances without supplemental oxygen.
2. Impaired memory R/T previous head injury M/B client stating some difficulty with short-term memory problems.
3. Chronic pain R/T back and pelvis injury M/B client stating he is in constant pain and experiences some physical immobility.

4. Impaired gas exchange R/T history of smoking and COPD M/ B requiring oxygen to walk longer distances and during the night, and he complains of not being able to breathe well.

Self-Assessment. *Comment on what you learned in the process of doing the interview. What are some of your interviewing strengths and what skills do you need to develop further?*

I found this interview to be very challenging because I had to interview a complete stranger about some very personal issues and beliefs. I have never been in a situation quite like the wellness interviews, and that is what makes it even more challenging. As we discussed after the interview, I tend to ask more direct questions. This worked out satisfactorily with B.W., as he seemed comfortable with my interviewing style. He answered almost all my questions and was open to discussion on many issues.

Now, when I think about the interview, I can see how asking direct questions would not work well with all types of people. I would like to work on the skill of question asking in order to be comfortable asking direct, indirect, and open-ended questions, because not all clients will be as comfortable talking as B.W. was. I would also like to work on not thinking about my next question while the client is talking. I found myself doing this when I was searching for a question to get at the topic of his support network. I wanted to find out more about how his relationship with his girlfriend related to his support and his ability to be there to support someone else.

I got distracted trying to think of a good way to find out that information. I think I did a good job at rephrasing my questions when B.W. didn't understand what I was asking. I also tried using silence to allow him to think about the issue and add more information if he wanted to. In some instances, he would use the silence and would explore the topic more, but other times I would then move on to a new question if I felt that he wasn't going to add anything. I feel I was able to hide my nervousness well and was able to make my interviewee feel comfortable and relaxed during our conversation.

Overall, it was a positive experience. I don't think I would choose to do it over again, but I was happy that I accomplished an interview in front of my peers with someone I had never met before—I knew it would be a challenge. I was pleased to learn that I really could ask the questions I have always considered to be the difficult ones.

SAMPLE 2

Interviewer: Student 2   Date: 3-25-03
Interviewee: Susan   Marital Status: Single
Age: 44   Gender: Female

Wellness
The interview failed to get Susan's definition of wellness. This was mostly due to the fact that Susan was every "closed down." When asked her definition of wellness, she responded, "I'm 40% well." She said that she is 40% well because she is able to get out of bed in the morning and function at some level. Though this did not answer the question directly, the rest of the interview gave clues as to what Susan's definition of wellness actually was. Susan seemed to focus on her physical health problems the most, but it was obvious that she was also dealing with mental, social, and spiritual issues as well. These topics will be discussed in detail further in the paper.

Physical
Susan is a 44-year-old female who is currently battling with ovarian cancer. She was diagnosed in December of 2002 and was hospitalized for nearly 7 months. Because of her physical health problems, she walks with a cane. Susan stated that using the cane was a major challenge in everyday life. She is obese and has a history of substance abuse. She seems to focus on her physical health problems, and this seems to carry over and cause problems with her mental, social, and spiritual health. Throughout the interview, Susan spoke in a very quiet voice. She maintained eye contact at times, and seemed to get teary-eyed at times during the interview. When asked questions about her cancer, Susan smirked and seemed annoyed at times. This was probably a defense mechanism in order to push me away.

Mental
Susan's mental status is appropriate in the areas of judgment, concrete thinking, and abstract thinking. I came to this conclusion because she was able to follow the conversation without becoming confused. Her responses were appropriate. Her speech was clear and at an appropriate tempo. The conversation had a logical flow, considering that Susan's mood was one of hopelessness and despair. She spoke in a very soft

voice and admitted that she was depressed. She had a "why me" attitude about her cancer.

Social
Susan has very little social support. She claimed she didn't want to get close to anyone because of her illness. She thinks that since she might die from the cancer, it is not worth making friends or having social relationships. Susan said the cancer "is my problem" and that she doesn't want to burden other people with her problems. Susan's mother is not a support for her because her mother is certain that Susan is going to die and is very emotional. Susan feels as though she is her mother's support, not that her mother supports her. This is very burdensome for Susan, because she says she doesn't want people to be concerned about her. When asked about past relationships, Susan said that in the past she had people close to her, but none of the relationships were healthy. Since she doesn't rely on others for support, Susan watches TV (football is her favorite), plays games on the Internet, and reads in order to relax. She is also taking classes at MATC. This helps her get her mind off of the cancer and keeps her busy. Susan understands that she is not coping well and doesn't think that she will be able to cope better in the future. She said that she isn't coping with the cancer any better now than she was when she was first diagnosed. Overall it is obvious that Susan is trying to isolate herself socially to avoid having feelings toward other people. It definitely seems as though she wants a friend or someone to talk to—she just doesn't know how to go about doing it.

Spirit
When asked about spirituality, Susan said that there is a higher power. She believes that "things happen for a reason." In regard to her cancer, she is still not sure as to what the reasons for it are. She takes life "day by day." Susan said that spirituality helps her get through her daily life, but she didn't specify as to exactly how spirituality helps her or what she does that is spiritual.

Goals/Future
Susan said that she really doesn't have any goals for the future because she is "not sure how long she is going to be here." Susan later said that she would like to finish school at MATC, but she didn't think that this was a realistic goal because she was dying.

Nursing Diagnoses

1. Activity intolerance related to sedentary lifestyle, manifested by inability to perform activities.
2. Anxiety related to threat to physical integrity, manifested by feelings of helplessness and discomfort.
3. Compromised family coping related to overwhelming situation regarding ovarian cancer and death of brother/son, manifested by abandonment and disregard for the patient's needs.
4. Ineffective coping related to diagnosis of cancer, manifested by verbalization of inability to cope, history of substance abuse, and social isolation.
5. Fear related to threat of death manifested by denial.
6. Hopelessness related to prolonged isolation and terminal/chronic illness manifested by social isolation and inability to set goals.

Self-Assessment

I found this interview to be very difficult. I felt very uncomfortable throughout the interview. I didn't know what to say in response to her hopeless and depressed attitude. I tried to give Susan time to think and expand on her answers; however, it seemed that she wasn't very interested in talking with me. I understand that she is a very closed down and reserved person; however, I feel that I should have been able to open her up more than I did. If I could do the interview over, I would try to establish a more relaxed conversation at first. A good opportunity to do this would have been to talk casually about football for a few minutes. Doing this would have calmed my nerves and possibly made Susan more comfortable. This would have taken the focus off of her physical health problems for a few minutes. I would also have asked her what she wanted to get out of the interview.

After the interview was over and I had time to think about it, it was obvious that Susan wanted someone to talk to. Had I asked this question, Susan may have opened up more. I think that I did a good job in asking open-ended questions and giving her a chance to explain her feelings. I was not judgmental of her and tried to be supportive of her. I also tried to focus on positive things in her life so that the situation didn't seem as depressing as it actually was. I didn't want Susan to leave thinking that she was a failure or that there really was no hope for her. Overall, this was a great learning experience. I learned that there is not always a right answer or response to the patient; sometimes, it is just better to listen.

Sample Wellness Group Documentation

The students in each section collaborate to develop a plan for their group that provides a general overview and a more specific outline for each session. Most semesters, each student takes a turn being the leader, but a flu clinic during the semester when the following described group took place necessitated that two students share leadership responsibilities for the fifth session.

[**Note:** Information on the following samples was included with written consent of the involved students. All names have been changed to assure the anonymity of the students and residents.]

SAMPLE WELLNESS GROUP PLAN

Statement of purpose: To develop a sense of connectedness and community among the members of the group. To provide educational support related to wellness by using a holistic approach that includes body, mind, and spirit.

Rationale. Staff thought a men's wellness group would be beneficial based on the requests of the male residents at the Triangle.

Description of target population. Adult males age 18+.

Member Criteria: Any males who reside at the Triangle.

Guidelines for group participation:

1. Be courteous.

2. Follow social rules (don't talk when others are talking, don't disregard someone else's ideas, etc.)
3. Honor confidentiality.

Group format and structure. It depends—up to eight people in one group, split into two groups if necessary.

Session	Dates	Leader	Theme
1. Social	10/16	Sue	Introductions and orientation to men's wellness and wellness groups
2. Stress Reduction	10/23	Ben	Education of relaxation and stress reduction techniques
Flu Clinic	10/30	No group	
3. Physical Activity	11/6	Cindy	Finding ways to incorporate fitness into everyday activities
4. Nutrition	11/13	Liza	Increasing awareness of simple ways to incorporate healthy eating habits
5. Relationships	11/20	Leanne and Christa	How communication effects the development of relationships and intimacy
6. Spirituality	12/4	Brittany	Discuss various ways to cope

Session Overviews. Each leader needs to provide the following information for his/her particular session:

SESSION 1: ORIENTATION

1. Behavioral objective(s) for the session (i.e., what is to be accomplished in behavioral terms?).

    a. Build a trusting therapeutic relationship with and among the group members and students in order to facilitate open discussion and learning in this and future sessions

    b. Have group members participate in group discussions as a way of building a sense of community and connectedness

    c. Develop an understanding of our (student nurses) purpose at the Triangle and benefits of coming and participating in our future wellness sessions

2. Overview of the activities planned.

    a. Students will introduce themselves

    b. Everyone will help themselves to a beverage and a morning snack

    c. Group participants will introduce themselves and explain how they heard of our wellness groups

    d. Explain what we are doing at the Triangle and why we are doing a men's wellness group

    e. Discuss wellness by having the participants first share their thoughts and then discuss what ways we having been learning about wellness

    f. Discuss the goals and expectations of the group members (explore ideas for topics, what they need help with, and what they would want to learn more about)

    g. Discuss what our groups will be doing in the next few weeks: dates and times and places of the meetings in the next weeks

    h. Discuss what members need to know for the next week's session and where to look for our flyers

3. Intended benefit of the session for the physical, mental, social, and/ or spiritual of health: We hope this session will benefit our member by allowing them to increase their sense of community and initiate the construction of relationships and friendships between the Triangle residents.

4. Identification of any special arrangements or materials needed: We plan on providing beverages and snacks (coffee, juice, bagels, and fruit).

5. Evaluation of effectiveness.

    a. Observe participants' abilities to interact with others in the group

    b. Monitor participants throughout the first and consecutive sessions for increased ability to socialize

SESSION 2: STRESS MANAGEMENT

1. Goal of this session is to provide some relaxation during the course of our group meeting and to provide relaxation tools and techniques to the members to use in an ongoing basis for stress reduction and relaxation.
    a. Help members recognize persistent stressors, and have them identify how the stress makes them feel
    b. Encourage discussion and sharing of ideas on what members are currently doing to help relieve stress in their lives
    c. Have members' rate current stress level
    d. Teach deep breathing
    e. Go through visualization exercise
    f. Rate stress level after exercise
2. Overview of the activities planned.
    a. Start with fun activity of painting pumpkins. Get people talking and laughing: 15–20 minutes
    b. Discussion of stress. What it is for the members and how they deal with it: 20 minutes
    c. Play soft music. Teach deep breathing: 5 minutes
    d. Visualization exercise: 5 minutes
    e. Discussion of how they are feeling after exercise and answer any questions: 5–10 minutes
3. Intended benefit of the session for the physical, mental, social, and/ or spiritual of health.
    Benefits of stress reduction session will be to help individuals find a sense of balance and energy by finding ways to manage stress. Stress management promotes well being in all areas of health, from physical, mental, and social to spiritual.
4. Identification of any special arrangements or materials needed: relaxation tape, music, candles
5. Evaluation of effectiveness by means of a stress level survey before and after the relaxation exercise and through the discussion about stress and post exercise. Observation of members' moods.

SESSION 3: PHYSICAL FITNESS

1. Behavioral objectives: Each member will participate in the exercises, stretches, and skills demonstrated. Members will be asked to share their own exercises and stretches and demonstrate to the group.

One goal is to have everyone find a skill that they will continue to use outside of the group.

2. Overview of activities planned: Activities will include demonstrations of muscle strengthening exercises, demonstrations of stretching, ROM, education about importance of activity for health, opportunities to share individual experiences, ideas for incorporating fitness activities into everyday life, modified exercises for those in wheel chairs, ways to make exercise fun.
3. Intended benefits
   a. Physical: to improve physical fitness and muscle strength
   b. Mental: to gain awareness of benefits of exercise, to reduce stress
   c. Social: to increase interaction of the group and share wellness ideas with others
4. Special arrangements or materials: It may be beneficial to meet in the fitness room to demonstrate the use of the equipment. Also, I would like to do some arm exercises with weights or soup cans, depending on abilities.
5. Evaluation of Effectiveness: resident self-report.

SESSION 4: NUTRITION

1. Behavioral Objective: to encourage healthy eating patterns and habits.
2. Overview of Activities:
   a. The food pyramid
   b. Education on correct serving sizes (what they actually look like). I may bring a serving size of vegetables/fruit for each
   c. Recipe sharing/healthy recipes collection—maybe each nursing student can bring favorite healthy recipe to share
   d. Menu planning for one week
   e. Basic shopping list
   f. Shopping list of ADA recommended foods
   g. Supplements
3. Intended benefit of the session: Encouraging healthy eating patterns and habits by educating and providing information on how to use the food pyramid to determine portion sizes and establish a meal plan. How to shop for these meals and how to create meals designed for specific restricted diets.

4. Identification of any special arrangements: prepare sample foods and serving sizes.
5. Evaluation for effectiveness will be through group participation, discussion, and demonstration.

SESSION 5: RELATIONSHIPS AND INTIMACY

1. Behavioral objectives for session.
   a. Learn appropriate ways to initiate conversation
   b. Discuss what is appropriate to share in conversation
   c. Learn effective ways to end a conversation
2. Overview of activities.
   a. All residents and students will introduce themselves.
   b. Residents and students will discuss the rules of conversation.
   c. Residents and students will play the conversation game.
3. Intended benefit of the session: Residents and students will construct the building blocks to form a strong relationship bridge. We hope this session will benefit the residents by facilitating effective communication techniques enabling them to increase their sense of connectedness in community.
4. Identification of any special arrangements/materials. We will need colored paper, markers, something to throw, tape, paper easel, and treats.
5. Evaluation of effectiveness will be through residents discussing the rules of conversation and playing the conversation game.

SESSION 6: SPIRITUALITY

1. Behavioral objectives for the session.
   a. Members will discuss how they currently cope
   b. Discussion will be held on different mechanisms of coping
   c. Community resources will be provided, such as support groups etc.
2. Overview of Activities.
   a. Provide overview of the day's information, including definition of coping
   b. Discussion by group of ways they currently use coping mechanisms

    c.   Information provided by leader on other mechanisms of coping

    d.   Community resources will be presented

3. Intended benefit of the session.

    a.   Current coping mechanisms will be further developed

    b.   New coping mechanisms will be presented

    c.   Awareness will be made of community resources

4. Identification of special arrangements or materials needed.

    a.   List of community resources

    b.   Healthy snacks

5. Evaluation of effectiveness will be made through feedback from members about the information provided and questions asked during the group. Members will also state how further development of current coping techniques and new coping mechanisms can be used in daily life.

Each student takes a turn being the group recorder and writing a group progress note on a standardized form. During the debriefing, the recorder shares his or her findings and documents further observations from the other participants. The instructor collects the form each week to evaluate the recorder's ability to document group content and process. The completed forms are returned to the student group at the end of the semester to facilitate their writing a summary of the overall group.

SAMPLE WELLNESS GROUP PROGRESS NOTE

Recorder: Date:

List all participants in attendance (identify whether student, staff, patient, resident, etc.)

Identify roles each played For the leader also identify the leadership style.

_____

_____

_____

_____

Provide evidence or examples . . .

_____

That the overarching group goal(s) are being met.

State the goal(s):

That the goal(s) for this session
are being met.

State the goal(s).

Of barriers to achievement of
goals.

Of group norms.

Check any of Yalom's therapeutic factors that were evident in the group, and give specific examples to support their presence.

Therapeutic factor	Evidence that factor was present
Imparting of information	
Catharsis: getting it all out	
Development of socialization skills	
Interpersonal learning: transfers to other situations	
Imitative behavior: identification with healthier members	
Corrective recapitulation: resolution of early conflicts with primary group	
Group cohesiveness: sense of solidarity, bonding	
Universality: knowing one is not alone	
Instillation of hope: seeing others who have triumphed	
Altruism: helping self by helping others	
Existential factors: establishing meaning	

Comment on what went particularly well in the group and what needs to be worked on:

SAMPLE LEADERSHIP SUMMARIES

After taking on the leadership role each student reflects on his/her experience by responding to five questions. The questions are apparent in the following summaries of the two students who co-led the fifth session of the previously described Men's Wellness Group.

Leanne

1. *Briefly describe the theme and activities for your session.* The theme of the session was communication. The activities planned were discussing the rules of conversation, playing the conversation game with the bunny, and discussing the building blocks to a strong relationship by building a rainbow (this last activity did not happen).

2. *Describe your leadership style.* I like control. If I had led the group by myself, I think the outcome would have not been as good because, instead of letting the group members talk about what they deemed important, I would have been trying to fit everything in. Thankfully, Christa was there to ground me and remind me of the bigger goal with the group—namely, getting them to communicate effectively.

3. *In what way were group goals met or advanced the in your session?* The overall goal is to build connectedness in community. The residents were given time to express themselves in a neutral situation. They were able to model the behavior we were trying to elicit by simply having a conversation. They learned to validate and repeat things that others said. All of these things are tied into connectedness within community.

4. *Identify what went well.* Individuals in the group were able to express things that are important to them. They were able to talk about what they like about conversation, whether it be humor, attentive listening, or a sense of understanding. The group got to witness Christa and me struggling a bit to get things going at times, but they saw us work effectively together through good communication. We modeled what we were trying to get the residents to learn. One personal thing that went well was my not appearing anxious. I was sweating a bit, but my voice didn't shake, and I wasn't talking fast, as I usually do, Yeah!

5. *Identify what could be improved.* I thought the organization could have been a bit better. Though Christa and I knew what we wanted to do, the game got confusing and had to be revamped during the group. It turned out that the residents got to see us interact and communicate to come up with something different, but I would have liked to have had it work the first time. Also, we planned too much for the given time. We didn't get to our last activity.

My own personal thing that needs improvement is learning what to say in those awkward situations. Christa seemed to know what to say but didn't say it. I, on the other hand, wanted to get a bit defensive and then draw the resident out to talk about it. I need to do a better job of owning my feelings.

Christa

1. *Briefly describe the theme and activities for your session.* Our session's theme was communication and relationships. We chose three activities, which were (1.) brainstorming good communication skills, (2.) the conversation game, and (3.) building a bridge to a strong relationship.
2. *Describe your leadership style.* My leadership style during the group worked toward facilitation of conversation more than leading. Leanne and I agreed that a lecture format would not work well with this topic because communication is different for everyone. We thought that allowing the group to lead itself at times would be more helpful in practicing communication with others. I tried to keep everyone involved by giving them all the chance to talk and express himself or herself.
3. *In what way were group goals met or advanced the in your session?* Our goals were met by the group's conversing openly. Even though there were some instances of inappropriate comments, the group was able to work through some of them and move on, such as was exemplified by Joe's comment to Gilbert. I think one aspect in which communication could have improved was Dave's comments about the nursing students, which seemed fake. I should have asked or tried to clarify what he said.
4. *Identify what went well.* I think the session allowed many of the participants to share their thoughts and feelings, which was good

for everyone because we saw different perspectives from people, and it showed personality traits of individuals that our group had not seen before. I'm glad that we did not try to fit in our last activity because I do not think it would have fit with the direction the group went.

5. *Identify what could be improved.* I think we could have improved many things about the group. I, personally, am still learning to interject in conversation. There was a point during the group when Leanne and I wanted to move on, neither of us could interrupt appropriately. I also think we could have put more planning into the group. When our game did not work, we both were pretty upset about it, even though it worked out to benefit the group.

At the end of the semester, each clinical section of students collaborates to compose a brief summary of the six sessions of their group.

SAMPLE WELLNESS GROUP SUMMARY

Students: Sue, Ben, Cindy, Liza, Leanne, Christa, and Brittany

1. *Name and location of the group:* Men's Wellness Group at the Triangle.
2. *Group purpose.* Our purpose was to develop a sense of connectedness and community among the members of the group and to provide educational support related to wellness by using a holistic approach including body, mind and spirit.
3. *Group goals, including whether and how they were met.*
    a. Develop community and relations between members and community as evidenced by group participation and use of skills developed in group
    b. Educational goals were met through demonstration of feedback in groups by members of information discussed and demonstration of understanding in terms of wellness.
4. *Group structure.*
    a. Membership criterion: Any males who reside at the Triangle
    b. Number of sessions and dates the group met. Six groups met on Thursdays, starting on 10/16/03 and ending on 12/04/03, with no group meeting on 10/30/03 due to a flu clinic
    c. List the theme and key activities of each session

- Session 1: Getting to know each other-introductions, explain purpose of group, discuss goals of groups, discuss wellness, discuss goals for group members, and discuss future groups
- Session 2: Stress reduction—pumpkin painting, discussion of stress, deep breathing, soft music, visualization, benefits of stress reduction
- Session 3: Physical Activity—stretches, exercises, members share exercise ideas, demonstrations of ROM, ideas for incorporating exercise into everyday life, play a game
- Session 4: Nutrition—discuss food pyramid, serving size demo, shopping list for food pyramid, how much fiber? Supplement matching, discussion of healthy eating habits
- Session 5: Communication—communication game, discussion of how to talk to people, what is or isn't appropriate to share with someone that you just met
- Session 6: Spirituality—provide overview of day's information, discuss current coping mechanisms, what does spirituality mean to you? Sharing of community resources, ending of groups

d. Provide a summary attendance list that includes the name of all the participants and the number of times they attended.

Joe	4	Tim	4	Warren	2
Gilbert	6	Micky	1	George	2
Dave	4	Charlie	3	James	2
Greg	5	Ron	5	Stan	2
Keith	6	Bill	1		

5. *Developmental phase of the group at its conclusion.* Our group reached the final or termination phase as evidenced by individual members verbalizing what the group had meant to them.

6. *Leadership styles.*
   Autocratic leaders focus on themselves and generally have the idea that their way is best. These groups have high productivity but low morale. Democratic leaders focus on members and members are encouraged to give input to all issues. Productivity is lower than in autocratic groups but morale is much higher. Laissez-faire style leaders have no focus and no input from a leader. Productivity and morale are very low.

   Sue: Democratic—asked group members what they would like to gain from wellness groups.

ȷen: Democratic—invited people to share feelings about stress.

Cindy: Democratic—members were encouraged to participate fully. Took suggestions from group members about how to change-up games.

Liza: Democratic—Provided members with hands-on samples of food and offered lots of choices so that members could choose what would work for them in their lives.

Leanne & Christa: Democratic—worked as a team to play a game. When it didn't work out as planned, received input from members on how to improve game.

Brittany: Democratic—allowed group to flow in direction that group wanted to go, with input at crucial points.

7. *Give some examples of group norms* apparent throughout the whole experience and discuss how they were developed (formally or informally): We were flexible in time—allowed members to come and go as they pleased—developed informally. When group members were holding the object of the day, that member knew that it was his turn to talk, and other members did not talk at the same dime—this developed informally.

8. *Roles:*

   a. *Identify some of the client roles and provide examples of behaviors that made them apparent. Were client roles fixed or flexible?*

   Resident roles were consistent and fairly fixed:

   Ron: *Comedian,* who provided comic relief with jokes and one-liners of wisdom. Sometimes a *monopolizer* in that he would talk over other group members.

   Dave: *Encourager,* who shared thoughts and insights.

   Greg: *Encourager,* who was especially insightful and who added to the cultural fullness of the group.

   Keith: *Blocker,* who randomly added comments that were inappropriate at times

   Warren: Monopolizer and, at times, *seducer* who shared intimate details that made others uncomfortable.

   Tim: *Mute,* who often sat quietly and usually left early.

b. *Each student needs to identify at least one role she or he played in the group beyond that of leader and give an example of how the role was manifested.*

Ben: *Initiator,* who keep things moving when group was quiet or slow and who was a *harmonizer* when he intervened in squabble with Greg and Keith.

Cindy: *Information recorder* when she wrote down members' ideas to assist peer leaders, and *follower,* as evidenced by her being an often passive participant who listened intently to group interactions.

Sue: *Coordinator,* who often clarified group ideas and brought relationships together to help gain a greater understanding of group.

Christa: *Gatekeeper,* who often paid attention to which group members had not said anything or had not participated and encouraged those members to participate if necessary.

Leanne: *Encourager,* who often recognized qualities of group members and promoted acceptance of group members' ideas.

Liza: *Energizer,* who motivated peer group members to perform at higher level of energy, often with humor and a high level of excitement.

Brittany: *Elaborator,* who expanded on group ideas and offered unique perspectives on group plans and objectives.

9. *Which of Yalom's therapeutic factors were most evident in the group? Give examples of group occurrences that support the contention that they were regularly present: for example, high group cohesiveness, members shared feelings about various topics, entire participation from group when sharing occurred.* Everyone participated in all groups to their fullest extent possible for that day.

10. *Recommendations for future groups.* Further groups should continue to develop communication and relationships. Also, recognition of group members who evidenced limitations and, in recognizing them, provision of accommodations to those members so as not to limit their involvement.

Clinical Evaluation Tools

Each component (Medical-Surgical and Psychosocial-Spiritual) has a standardized clinical evaluation tool (CET) that documents student progress in relation to the course objectives. Instructors enter comments that are shared on a regular basis with students to keep them informed of their strengths and areas for further development. The students add their comments to their CETs during formal reviews at midterm and the end of the semester. Completed CETs are signed by each involved instructor and student and forwarded to the student's academic advisors.

PSYCHOSOCIAL-SPIRITUAL COMPONENT CLINICAL EVALUATION TOOL TEMPLATE

Clinical Evaluation Tool   Student:

Psycho-Social-Spiritual Health   Advisor:

Instructor: Semester:

CLINICAL OBJECTIVES

1. **Health.** Uses *nursing process* to structure holistic care for clients.
2. **Environment.** Advocates effectively for *continuity of care* and a continuum of services.
3. **Client.** *Collaborates* with assigned clients and other care providers to assure high quality care.
4. **Professional nursing.** Demonstrates *commitment and accountability* in clinical practice.

5. **Caring.** Develops self as a *therapeutic agent* who respects rights and individuality of each client.
6. **Critical thinking.** *Applies theoretical knowledge* (related to mental illness and psycho-social-spiritual intervention) to clinical practice with clients experiencing chronic illness.

Rating key: Meets the standard (✓), Exceeds the standard (+), Fails to meet the standard (−)

Each assignment or critical behavior is considered essential and must be satisfactorily demonstrated to pass the course. Passing the course includes satisfactory completion of the following:

OUTCOME MEASURES	Date	Rating (− ✓ +) and Instructor Comments
Dass & Gorman Chapters 1–8		
Interview & Written Summary		
Interview Notes		
Group Plan		Done as a group
Group Progress Note		
Group Leadership Summary		
Group Summary		Done as a group
Independent Experiences		
Professionalism		Attendance, punctuality, special contributions

Midterm Evaluation

Student Comments (See Blackboard for guidelines)   **Date:**
Instructor Comments and Midterm Rating: **Date:**

Final Evaluation

Student Comments (See Blackboard for guidelines)   **Date:**
Instructor Comments and Final Rating: **Date:**

Instructor Signature: _____ Date: _____

Student Signature: _____ Date: _____

MEDICAL-SURGICAL COMPONENT CLINICAL EVALUATION TOOL TEMPLATE

Clinical Evaluation Tool Template for Med/Surg. Component

Course Description: Managing nursing care with individuals and families experiencing complex, long-term health problems. Emphasis on multidisciplinary collaborative planning and continuity of care.

Student: _____ **Semester:** _____

Clinical Area: _____ **Instructor:** _____

Final Course Grade: _____

I am willing to have subsequent clinical instructors review this evaluation for the purpose of promoting my learning in future clinical experiences.

Student Signature: _____

Students are responsible for completing the evaluation form prior to each conference with faculty. Student and faculty will collaborate in the evaluation process. Faculty have final responsibility for assigning course grade. Student and faculty conference is a desired (but not required) outcome.

Each critical behavior is considered essential and must be satisfactorily demonstrated to pass the course. Passing the course includes satisfactory completion of all the assignments.

Evaluation Standards

Fails to meet the standard: (−)

- Demonstrates expected behavior only occasionally or inconsistently

- Requires promoting or reminders from others to initiate executed behaviors
- Requires assistance from others to demonstrate the behavior
- Seldom initiates expected behavior
- Performs expected behavior inaccurately or incompletely
- Makes errors in performance and/or judgment, or would make errors without the interventions of others
- Does not recognize need for assistance and/or does not request assistance when needed
- Performance is not significantly improved with practice and experience
- Often fails to solve simple problems or make routine clinical decisions

Meets the standard: (✓)

- Demonstrates expected behavior consistently
- Initiates expected behaviors constantly
- Requests assistance as needed and appropriate
- Rarely requires reminders to demonstrate expected behavior
- Demonstrate competence in expected behavior
- Performance improves with practice and experience
- Consistently solves routine problems
- Makes accurate clinical decisions in routine situations

Exceeds the standard: (+)

- Demonstrate mastery of expected behaviors
- Arrives at creative solutions to complex or non-routine problems
- Seeks additional experiences and interactions to enhance knowledge and skill beyond the expected behaviors for the course in a professional and appropriate manner
- Anticipates needs of clients and/or staff, and takes action appropriately to meet needs
- Requires no prompting, reminders or assistance to demonstrate expected behaviors
- Level of performance is consistent across time

HEALTH

Program Outcomes: Demonstrate critical thinking skills and caring practices to promote, maintain, and restore health.

Course Objectives(CO)/Essential Criteria	Midterm			Final		
	Fails	Meets	Exceeds	Fails	Meets	Exceeds
CO1. Apply the nursing process to maximize the functioning of adults with chronic illness						

- Collects data that is pertinent and relevant for the client
- Analyzes data that includes the client's abilities as well as health needs
- Establishes realistic outcomes based on data analysis
- Selects nursing interventions designed to promote client's functioning
- Evaluates effectiveness of nursing care in terms of outcome achievement and client/family satisfaction

Evaluated by:
Weekly clinical prep sheets
Participation in student conference on the unit
Observation of clinical practice

Comments—Midterm Evaluations:

Comments—Final Evaluation:

ENVIRONMENT

Program Outcomes: Respond to environmental factors that influence the health of individuals, families, and communities.

Course Objectives/Essential Criteria	Midterm			Final		
	Fails	Meets	Exceeds	Fails	Meets	Exceeds
CO2. Advocates for needed resources to assure continuity of care.						

- Identifies client's needs for continued care
- Develops a plan to facilitate continuity of care as the client changes settings

Evaluated by:
Discharge planning issues discussed in weekly clinical prep
Attends rehab activities

Comments—Midterm Evaluation:

Comments—Final Evaluation:

CLIENT

Program Outcomes: Collaborate with clients and colleagues in the process of identifying and organizing resources for the effective provision of health care.

Course Objectives/Essential Criteria	Midterm			Final		
	Fails	Meets	Exceeds	Fails	Meets	Exceeds
CO3. Collaborate with multidisciplinary team to promote client participation in treatment.						

- Makes meaningful contributions to treatment planning by the multidisciplinary team
- Integrates nursing interventions with strategies of other health team members
- Interacts with health team members in a collegial manner

Evaluated by:
Participation in multidisciplinary team meetings or discharge planning
Observation of clinical practice

Comments—Midterm Evaluation:

Comments—Final Evaluation:

PROFESSIONAL NURSING

Program Outcomes: Demonstrate professional behaviors that reflect accountability and commitment in nursing practice.

Course Objectives/Essential Criteria	Midterm			Final		
	Fails	Meets	Exceeds	Fails	Meets	Exceeds
CO4. Demonstrate commitment and accountability for clinical decision making.						

- Maintains ethical standards of professional behavior
- Protects client information while sharing needed data to promote continuity of care
- Critique own decision making to improve nursing practice

Evaluated by:
Weekly written self evaluation
Weekly journal entries
Attendance, punctuality, professional attire
Accountability
Preparation
Application of Code of Ethics

Comments—Midterm Evaluation:

Comments—Final Evaluation:

CARING

Program Outcomes: Establish therapeutic relationships with clients that demonstrate caring.

Course Objec- tives/Essential Criteria	Midterm			Final		
	Fails	Meets	Exceeds	Fails	Meets	Exceeds
CO5. Develop self as therapeutic agent while maintaining respect for client individuality.						

- Adapts nursing care in a manner that is respectful of client individuality
- Identifies the client/family point of view regarding health care needs
- Interactions with clients/families regardless of personal beliefs

Evaluated by:
Observation of clinical practice
Weekly journal entries

Comments—Midterm Evaluation:

Comments—Final Evaluation:

CRITICAL THINKING

Program Outcome: Synthesize knowledge from nursing theory, research and practice, the humanities, and the natural and behavioral sciences to provide a basis for professional nursing practice.

Course Objectives/Essential Criteria	Midterm			Final		
	Fails	Meets	Exceeds	Fails	Meets	Exceeds
CO6. Make clinical decisions that reflect consideration of context.						

- Makes clinical decisions that reflect context while maintaining standards of practice
- Adapts nursing care to meet health care needs within the context of the client's environment

Evaluated by:
Teaching/Learning project
Clinical decision making
Medication Exam

Comments—Midterm Evaluation:

Comments—Final Evaluation:

Signatures

Date of Midterm Evaluation: _____ Student: _____ Instructor: _____
Date of Final Evaluation: _____ Student: _____ Instructor: _____

Sample Completed
Clinical Evaluation Tools

SAMPLE PSYCHOSOCIAL-SPIRITUAL COMPONENT CLINICAL EVALUATION TOOL

Clinical Evaluation Tool　　　　**Student:** Louise Shank
Psycho-Social-Spiritual Health　　**Advisor:** Jean Faculty
Instructor:　　　　　　　　　　　**Semester:** Fall 2003

CLINICAL OBJECTIVES (continued from Appendix D)

1. **Health.** Uses *nursing process* to structure holistic care for clients
2. **Environment.** Advocates effectively for *continuity of care* and a continuum of services
3. **Client.** *Collaborates* with assigned clients and other care providers to assure high quality care
4. **Professional nursing:** Demonstrates *commitment and accountability* in clinical practice
5. **Caring.** Develops self as a *therapeutic agent* who respects rights and individuality of each client
6. **Critical thinking.** *Applies theoretical knowledge* (related to mental illness and psycho-social-spiritual intervention) to clinical practice with clients experiencing chronic illness

Rating key: Meets the standard: (✓), Exceeds the standard: (+), Fails to meet the standard: (−)

Each assignment or critical behavior is considered essential and must be satisfactorily demonstrated to pass the course. Passing the course includes satisfactory completion of the following:

OUTCOME MEASURES	Date	Rating (– ✓ +) and Instructor Comments
Dass & Gorman Chapter 1	9/3	✓Thoughtful, honest response highlighting importance of balance between openness and sound boundaries.
Chapters 2 & 3	9/10	✓Identified commonalities between herself and the residents she'll be working with. Shared a recent military experience that illustrates her ability to accept help.
Chapter 4	9/24	✓+Honest assessment of need to listen beyond assumptions and surface characteristics of the clients.
Chapters 5 & 6	10/23	++Very detailed discussion of how she has opened up and thus stereotypes she held of people who were poor or mentally ill have been transformed. Louise did a superior job of applying what she has learned from assigned readings in both NRS 340 and 341 to the question at hand, and of providing examples of high profile legal cases that have helped to diminish stigmatized views of disability.
Chapters 7 & 8	10/29	+Very thoughtful discussion of importance of self care & maintaining individual identify to prevent burnout.
Interview	9/18	✓Interviewed 49-year-old male with incomplete spinal cord injury (SCI). Had difficulty containing her emotional distress over his situation as evidenced by being tearful throughout much of the interview. Was able to keep her focus on the resident and

		regroup enough to ask some meaningful questions. During debriefing, recognized that having taken care of several young adults with similarly incapacitating injuries earlier in the week without time to process the impact of the experience led to her difficulty today. Was very open to need to examine own values and how they might be inadvertently imposed on clients. Responded exceptionally well to constructive criticism exceptionally well and identified steps she'll take to enhance future interactions with Triangle residents. Took the initiative to follow up with the resident to assure that he was okay with the interview, and he assured her that he was.
Written Summary	9/19	✓Completed write-up in a very timely fashion. Documented relevant data as presented by client, although more examples to support her assessments would enhance the summary. Her ability to identify two meaningful nursing diagnoses suggests an adequate grasp of nursing process, but I encourage Louise to focus on diagnoses reflecting the client's strengths (e.g., spiritual well being) as well as limits. She completed a very candid and honest self-assessment that indicates openness to learning and a realistic sense of important areas for development (e.g., overcoming assumptions to minimize potential projection of own feelings on others, listening more deeply).
Interview Notes	9/11	✓+Notes on instructor-led interviews evidence good ability to collect rele-

		vant and meaningful data, organize it into domains of health, and substantiate resident concerns with direct quotes.
	9/18	+Documentation evidences that Louise makes very astute observations about the clients being interviewed.
	9/25	+Notes provide excellent guidance for student who will be writing up the interviews she's observed. Louise includes diagnostic formulations and advice to peers in her notes.
	10/2	✓+Provides meaningful data. Advice to peer especially helpful.
Group Plan Done as a group	10/8	+Louise worked collaboratively with her peers to develop an exceptionally complete and clearly delineated plan for a Men's Wellness Group. The students have done a superb job of identifying realistic objectives for each session and specifying how they will assess the effectiveness of the group. Louise's session will focus on increasing awareness of simple ways to incorporate healthy eating habits.
Group Progress Note	10/23	+Although she did not have the standard progress note form available, Louise took exceptionally thorough notes on today's group. She did an excellent job of documenting both the group content and process.
Group Leadership	11/13	+Led the 4th session of the Men's Wellness Group that was exceptionally well thought-out. Louise clearly articulated her intention, both in her written plan and in the group session (encouraging healthy eating behavior). She presented what can be

		rather staid information in a creative and engaging manner and did a super job of responding effectively to resident questions. Her strategy for conveying serving sizes was especially clever and served to promote participant interaction as well as to educate them. Louise presented with a confident and competent demeanor through the session in spite of her report during the debriefing that she was a little anxious and felt she went too fast. Her peers gave her much positive feedback regarding her ability to keep the group flowing and to convey some very valuable information. Her deep insight into group process and the importance of attending to the overall group purpose was in evidence when she wisely opted to promote participant sharing over lecturing about nutrition.
Written Summary	11/20	✓Completed written summary that provided adequate overview of the activity she designed and her role as the leader. Did a good job identifying how the session advanced the overall group goals.
Group Summary Done as a group	12/14	+Collaborated with peers to complete a very clear, concise, and thorough summary of the Men's Wellness Group. The report was exceptionally well organized and provided a superb delineation of the key roles many of the participants played over the course of the six sessions. Its value extends beyond the limits of the course as it will be used to help document the important work the students did in collaboration with the

		Triangle Community Ministry Parish (the "Triangle") nurse.
Independent Experiences	9/18	✓Spent **2.5** hours with Joy Drummond in the Triangle Foot Clinic.
	9/21	Completed a summary that included a general overview of the services provided at the Clinic and some good insights about the importance of listening.
	9/27	+Spent **2.5** hours at the VA Residential Substance Abuse Program on 9/25. Write-up provided a detailed description of the activities she engaged in and the various services provided by the program.
	10/14	+Completed her Independent Experience assignment by spending **2** hours on the TRU unit at Mendota. Provided a very thorough write-up that described the program and included a good mental status assessment for one patient she observed. Louise also did a good job identifying nursing roles in evidence there.
Professionalism	12/5	+Has not missed any clinical time and always punctual. Presents with a warm, friendly demeanor and has done a superb job of matching that with a more clear sense of therapeutic boundaries. Has continually extended herself beyond the requirements of the course, thus assuring that her learning has been optimal.
Miscellaneous	10/30	+Administered a number of IM injections during the Triangle's annual flu vaccine using proper technique. Her previous experience with this skill allowed her to demonstrate effectively

for her peers and served to calm their anxiety. She evidenced a very calm and poised demeanor that also readily put the residents at ease.

Midterm Evaluation

Student Comments   **Date:** 10/8/03

1. In general, I find it easy to speak to just about anyone and can usually find something that we can connect on and discuss. I work well as part of a team and have met with my clinical group on several occasions to discuss various issues and projects. It is beneficial for me to get together with everyone and bounce ideas off of one and other. It helps with my learning process. I am having some trouble coming up with my strengths.

2. I am very emotional. I should concentrate more on keeping my emotions in check and listening to people objectively instead of subjectively. I like a good story and tend to get wrapped up in people's stories. I should focus more on the here and now instead of the past. It will help me more as a nurse to help patients focus on what they can do now to help themselves instead of what they should have/could have done. I feel that I sometimes have a tendency to speak without thinking . . . sometimes things come out the way that I didn't necessarily mean or maybe people understood them in a different way than what I had meant.

3. I would like to be able to listen to a resident and glean the necessary information from what they say in order to help them get at what they need. Maybe become a better information gatherer. Ask more pertinent questions. I would like to learn more about group dynamics.

Instructor Comments   **Date:** 10/9/03

Midterm Rating. Louise is currently meeting expectations for all course objectives. In fact, she is an especially effective team member who pitches in without being asked and offers meaningful feedback about how the group is doing. Her discussion of areas in which she hopes to develop speaks to her good insight and motivation to do her best. I agree that it will be helpful for her to reign in her emotional expression to some degree, but not the depth of her feeling—her compassion for others is a key strength.

Final Evaluation

Student Comments   **Date:** 12/5/03

How are you different as a result of your work at the Triangle or Mendota? I am more aware. I am more aware of my surroundings and pay closer attention to people. I don't have as many assumptions that I used to have. I try to think more before I speak. I am more forgiving, more understanding, more open-minded. I refrain from projecting my opinions, emotions, and feelings onto the client. I take care of myself because I know that that is the only way I can truly give good nursing care.

Identify how you have grown in relation to each of the six course objectives:

Health. *Uses nursing process to structure holistic care for clients:* It is difficult for me to answer these evaluation questions individually because I feel like I am so much part of a group in this clinical. It seems like we should be getting a group evaluation instead. We utilized the nursing process in every group session that we did. When planning for my group on nutrition, I assessed the learners. Who were they? What would they expect? What were my perceptions of their needs? I made a diagnosis of the group. I planned for our activities and outcomes. I implemented the group during my scheduled time and made changes as necessary. During our debriefing of the group, I evaluated how I think things went, and then everyone gave their own feedback on the group in general.

Environment. *Advocates effectively for continuity of care and a continuum of services:* As a group during our men's wellness sessions, we have kept the resident's informed of group expectations. Everyone knows that they should be quiet when it is someone's turn to talk. The residents know that they should be respectful of one and other and of us. The residents were informed when group would start and how long the sessions would last. They know when we will be done with the sessions.

Client. *Collaborates with assigned clients and other care providers to assure high quality care:* I keep people informed. It is better to let people know what they should expect in any interaction. I try to assess what a client expects to gain from a certain interaction or action. If you know what someone expects to accomplish or gain, then it is a lot easier to let them know if it is something attainable or something that is outlandish.

Professional nursing. *Demonstrates commitment and accountability in clinical practice:* Taking a page out of Pamela's book, I own what I do. If I feel like I've made a mistake I say it. I have arrived to every clinical prepared and on time. I love the clinical at the Triangle. I love the residents. I am happy to be there and be with the people there. My enthusiasm—or "bubbliness," as my interviewee called it—is not contrived. It is a genuine feeling that I get from being at the Triangle. If I tell a resident or a peer that I am going to do something, I do it. I like people to know that I am a reliable person and that I can be counted on if needed to come through.

Caring. *Develops self as a therapeutic agent who respects rights and individuality of each client:* I respect each client's privacy and do not discuss client's personal information outside of the academic setting. I think that in order to develop a mutual trust with the client, this is a must. I genuinely care about my clients and am happy when they are doing things that are beneficial to their health.

Critical thinking. *Applies theoretical knowledge to clinical practice with clients experiencing chronic illness:* Whenever residents of the Triangle would start to act outside of their "normal behavior," I would start to question what could be going on with this person. By applying the knowledge that I may have had about a person's condition and current circumstances, I could theorize about what may be going on physiologically or emotionally with someone.

When doing my nutrition group, I realized that we were getting off of the plan that I had established originally. However, the reason that we weren't moving on was because everyone was sharing his or her thoughts on nutrition. I realized that this was more important because it fit with our group's overall goal of developing community in the Triangle.

What advice do you have for future students to help them maximize their learning in this clinical? Stay positive. Emotions are contagious. Pay attention. Listen. Keep an open mind. Don't project your emotions on to your client.

Instructor Comments   Date: 12/5/03

Final Rating: Satisfactory for all objectives, with Louise exceeding expectations on a number of parameters as indicated on the outcome measures grid. I agree with her self-assessment above and applaud her ability to recognize her gifts. Louise is a highly motivated, self-directed learner who seeks out opportunities to challenge herself. She is an exceptionally thoughtful and cooperative team member who always pitches in without having to be asked. She has done a marvelous job of giving balanced, constructive feedback to her peers. Her capacity for introspection and active engagement with those she works with and serves is exceptional. Louise's commitment to the client population of concern in this clinical was evident not only each week in the course, but also when she spent 5 hours of her own time to assist with the Triangle Christmas party on 12/7/03.

Instructor Signature: _____ Date: _____

Student Signature: _____ Date: _____

COMPLETED EVALUATION TOOL
FOR MED/SURG. COMPONENT

Ms. Mary

Course Objective 1: Applies the nursing process to maximize the functioning of adults with chronic illness.
Collects data that is pertinent and relevant for the client.
Analyzes data that includes the client's abilities as well as health needs.
Establishes realistic outcomes based on data analysis.
Selects nursing interventions designed to promote client's functioning.
Evaluates effectiveness of nursing care in terms of outcome achievement and client/family satisfaction.

Throughout the semester, Mary has demonstrated excellent skill in utilizing the nursing process to care for clients and their families. Mary is exceptionally thorough in collecting appropriate data to safely care for her patients and families. She makes accurate assessments of her patients and families based on comprehensive data collection and is able to identify appropriate nursing diagnoses from her data collection. Mary is able to identify actual patient problems and potential problems along with appropriate nursing interventions to resolve and/or prevent the problems. Her ability to intervene along with her decision making as it relates to acute symptom management improved greatly throughout the semester. Her clinical prep sheets demonstrate a very good understanding of the entire nursing process. Her goals are appropriate and her evaluation statements accurate. Throughout the semester, Mary has developed an excellent understanding of whole person care as it relates to the hospice population.

Course Objective 2: Advocates for needed resources to assure continuity of care.
Identifies client's needs for continued care.
Develops a plan to facilitate continuity of care as the client changes settings.

Mary was able to work with the nurses from both the admission team and the in-home team. This, along with her experience in inpatient care, has provided an excellent opportunity to understand issues related to continuity of care. Mary is able to apply the nursing process as it relates to any of these three settings and has developed an excellent understanding of the issues clients and families face in each of these three settings. She has expanded her circle of care to include families in a more meaningful dialogue that enhances continuity of care.

Course Objective 3: Collaborates with multidisciplinary team to promote client participation in treatment.
Makes meaningful contributions to treatment planning by the multidisciplinary team.
Integrates nursing interventions with strategies of other health team members.
Interacts with health team members in a collegial manner.

Mary has regularly attended the weekly IDG meetings and makes meaningful contributions to the team. Other health team members view Mary as a colleague rather than as a student nurse. Throughout the semester, Mary worked with all the staff members, keeping them well informed of patient and family issues. Mary also worked with the case manager to observe this role. Mary has developed a keen sense of the importance of communication and team building and has worked very hard to develop her sense of confidence in interacting with other team members.

Course Objective 4: Demonstrates commitment and accountability for clinical decision-making.

Maintains ethical standards of professional behavior.
Protects client information while sharing needed data to promote continuity of care.
Critique own decision making to improve nursing practice.

Mary is extremely reliable and professional in class. She is punctual and dresses professionally, her behavior is professional, she gets work in on time. She is consistently well prepared to provide professional, safe care for her clients. She assumes responsibility for her own learning and looks information up prior to clinical. She is an extremely motivated learner and utilizes every experience to maximize her learning. She asks questions when she is uncertain and is always safe. She is mindful of issues related to confidentiality and privacy.

Course Objective 5: Develops self as therapeutic agent while maintaining respect for client individuality.
Adapts nursing care in a manner that is respectful of client individuality.
Identifies the client/family point of view regarding health care needs.
Interacts with clients/families regardless of personal beliefs.

Mary does an excellent job when working with her clients to involve them in decision making and maximizing client independence and participation in their care, as they and their families desire. She demonstrates caring practices in dealing with clients and families. Her weekly journal entries demonstrate a thoughtful understanding of the hospice population and the challenges this group faces. Throughout the semester, Mary has been challenged by a variety of clients and clinical situations that have provided the opportunity to grow as an individual. Mary is able to see the value in every learning situation, despite how difficult or uncomfortable it may seem at the time. She continues to grow professionally as new challenges arise. As Mary developed further confidence in her communication skills, she found she was able to ask the difficult questions and intervene in a therapeutic manner that reflected caring and concern.

Course Objective 6: Makes clinical decisions that reflect consideration of context.
Makes clinical decisions that reflect context while maintaining standards of practice.
Adapts nursing care to meet health care needs within the context of the client's environment.

Mary worked with the entire clinical group to instruct a group of nursing assistants in learning new skills. Mary is developing a comprehensive nursing knowledge base upon which to draw and is able to use information from previous clinical situations and apply it appropriately to new situations. Her problem-solving skills have greatly developed throughout the semester as she assumed more responsibility. Mary is able to make cogent clinical decisions that reflect the individual context of her client and family.

Adrian's Story: A Long Time Ago in a Galaxy Far, Far Away . . .

The year was 1981. My partner John and I were headed in to work a nightshift at UW Hospital, I had to work the entire shift with this upwardly mobile nurse named Colleen Pfeiffer. We were listening to Public Radio when a small story about "gay cancer" came over the air. Apparently, young, otherwise healthy gay men were getting Kaposi's Sarcoma (KS), a cancer found in middle-aged men in the Mediterranean. These men were grouped in New York and San Francisco. I had lived and played in San Francisco and Washington, DC, in the mid-70s, but figured I was about as far removed from there as I could get. We shrugged it off, but little did we know that it would change our lives forever.

The funny part of that is that John and I are again living together. Well, it's not really as funny as it is a testament to our commitment to take care of each other. We met in a bar I used to own; I think that was in the mid '70s, on a night I really didn't want to meet anyone. I think I said something to that effect to John, but somehow I ended up going over to his very busy apartment that night and talking to him over eggs at Spud Nuts on State the next morning. I started moving into his pad within weeks of our meeting. Obviously, we thought long and hard about nothing but our attraction to each other. From the start, we had difficulties over issues of control, and still do to this day. Somehow, we managed to ignore this and lived together as partners until I moved out the year I turned 30, and, even more amazing, we've remained friends and are still each other's support after nearly 30 years. I know that you are thinking that we are much too young to have spent 30 years being there for each other. So, I'll lie and say we met in preschool. Now we spend time traveling and avoiding each other.

John is a very important person in my life, and we do depend on each other for many things. We have a commitment to help each other in times of need and also in times that are just plain frightening. We tend to understand each other, but that doesn't mean that we always agree. At least, we agree to disagree. We also tend to look after one another and keep tabs on each other's health. It is also very comforting to know that we will understand when the other needs a bit more sleep or just can't manage the strength to get through the daily grind. Sometimes we just need another ear to listen to our complaints or fears or a bit of hand holding and comforting. It works well for both of us.

Fast forward to 1984, when I was working in the Medical ICU at UW as a monitor tech. Sometime in March, a young man was admitted to the ICU in respiratory distress. By now, it was suspected that there was an infectious agent causing pneumocystis carinii pneumonia (PCP) and KS, and it was also giving young men something called gay related immune deficiency syndrome (GRIDS). Paul had whatever this was. His partner, whom had no rights or privileges in the ICU, didn't realized that his bedridden ventilated partner was going to be dead in a matter of days. He had no right to know, according to anyone in a position of authority. I shuddered at the lack of human compassion surrounding me; these were health care professionals, right? He had lost their apartment and his job and had spent the last of their savings to buy a "honeymoon" trip to Hawaii. I don't think his partner was allowed to go to Paul's funeral. I had a sinking feeling things were going to get a lot worse before they got better. I very silently said to myself that something had to be done.

Sometime in the late summer, I was monitoring 45 patients on heart monitors spread all over the hospital and outlying towns that needed a discriminating eye kept on their patients. We got a call from administration saying a person that was flying from New York to San Francisco needed emergency admittance to the ICU; he most likely had GRIDS. He was wheeled into a room about an hour later. He had PCP. We never spoke; he died before the day shift got in. I shuddered at the thought of them/me being alone, scared, dying, and the very worst thing, shunned and avoided by everyone that could get away with it. I listened to the jokes, heard the snickers, and wanted to be somewhere else. I promised myself that I would never watch this happen to my brothers again. Boy, the things we promise ourselves.

Fall has always been my favorite time of year; this one would be different. Jerry came rolling into the ICU. It seemed he had crashed somewhere up on the pulmonary unit, and, to boot, he had that new thing called acquired immune deficiency syndrome (AIDS). People didn't live very long—weeks, days, hours, you name it—so there really wasn't a big need for long-term care or planning, and damn little time to even consider palliative treatment. As I recall, human immunodeficiency virus (HIV) hadn't been discovered, so transmission was thought to be possible by a myriad of avenues: anal sex, kissing, touching—and even being in the same room with—the infected person, using poppers, and exposure to cytomegalovirus (CMV), among others. I had to sit through an entire shift of the same old barrage of jokes and discrimination; they hit so close to home. Why so much hate? My shift was coming to an end, and I had this little monster in my brain reminding me that I had a promise to keep.

I saw my head nurse, and asked to have a bit of her time. I walked into her office, told her my disturbing observations and some of the awful things I had heard. Then I took all my nerves, rolled them into one big ball, and tossed it at her. I was going into Jerry's room—I was going to start an organization to deal with all these issues, and I didn't really care how she felt about it. I offered to quit my job that day, to be free to work at whatever it was I was going to create. Much to my surprise, she hugged me, wiped the tears off my face, and offered any assistance she could give me. What? Did I hear correctly?

I started putting on my spacesuit. A bit of history here: in order to enter a room occupied by someone with this disease, you had to wear gloves (preferably four), a hat, a scrub suit, a mask, an isolation gown, and, of course, those ever so fashionable paper booties. In addition, anything the patient touched or used needed to be destroyed, as was the case with paper and plastic, or sterilized if possible. I still believe that part of the thought was to sterilize the hell and sins out of things touched by those people as much as for sterilization. It was very much a gay disease. I remember hearing that one of the hardest things about getting AIDS was trying to convince friends and family members that you were either a Haitian, a prostitute, or an IV drug user, anything but Gay.

I had been watching staff physicians ask from the doorway if everything was okay. Jerry was being ventilated—what could he say? I walked up to his bed and asked him when he had last seen a face, and had he been touched recently? He looked at me with these incredibly blue eyes, tears welling up, and he just shrugged. I decided to risk my life, I pulled my mask down under my chin, pulled off my gloves, smiled my most fearless, yet fetching, smile, and touched his arm and face. I knew right then that I had just committed myself to helping in anyway

I could. As far as I knew, I had just exposed myself to one of the most infectious and deadly diseases ever. I told Jerry of my plans, and asked him what he thought about the name Madison AIDS Support Network (MASN for short). It was thumbs up, and I was off and on my way to one of the most incredible journeys of my life, one that I am still on today.

Jerry lived for about a year-and-a-half after diagnosis, which was unheard of in itself. He died December 17, a Saturday, the day we were going to celebrate Christmas together at his house. At the funeral, his mom Irene asked if she could adopt me, his sister accused me of just being in this to get his money and his things, and I was just so incredibly and profoundly sad and hurt.

Sometime during this experience with Jerry, I found out that I had it. Yup, I was HIV+. I was the founder, a volunteer, and a client of MASN. My good friend and co-President of the board of directors of MASN, Will, came along to my first appointment and took notes. He had told me that I wouldn't remember the gist of the conversation with the physician. Hell, I could remember anything, besides, how bad could it be? I wouldn't lose my memory for a couple of years yet. He later mailed the notes to me. I didn't remember much past the doctor's declaration of HIV/AIDS. I went home, and for about 3 days cried and looked out my window, then I read Will's letter to me. Seems I had agreed to surgery.

How would I tell friends and family? I called my sister and asked if she could come over and take me out, *alone!* I told her. We cried a lot together that night, and we drove around Madison for hours. She kept telling me I couldn't die; I was her best friend. I kind of had the same feelings about dying, but everybody that got it did die, and pretty quickly, too. That was about all that I could get in to or out of my mind.

For the next months, I kept going out to my parent's home with every intention of telling them, but each and every time, my sister knew that this was not the right time to tell them. So, I took it upon myself to just set them down and tell them. Mom cried, and Dad swore. I really can't remember the reactions of other family members; I had a couple of things on my mind. Well, I certainly felt better about the entire situation, but what was I putting my family through now?

I believe that there are certain things that keep me alive. If I get so much as a bad hangnail, my family is aware of it. In fact, my sister and mother would probably show up with chicken noodle soup and something to do until I felt better. If I don't call somebody in the family for a while, they know that I'm either sick or in love; either way, they're going to find out. Calling my family supportive is inadequate; my family is way more than that. They are there before I can ask, and if I had a partner, I would expect the same of them. They still like John and invite him out often. I also laugh a lot. I decided that I needed to find more things funny and really get rid of negative emotions. They'll kill you. I have succeeded in riding my life of grudges, for the most part. Now, I need more rest then I used to, so I rest more. It really is pretty simple. Just learn to say no to the things that can harm you emotionally or physically and do more of the things that make you feel good. I know, I know, I sound like an old hippie. Heck, I am an old hippie. Imagine that, I'm old!

At this time my niece was 1 year old, the right time to tell her didn't come for 16 more years. I had spoken at an educational program for area High Schools, we were discussing a play/tap show we had seen performed about the life and times of someone I knew, an ex of John's; afterwards some of the students got to quizzing me about my life. And one thing led to another. I soon discovered they were from my niece's school; in fact they were her friends and fellow swim teammates. I had to act fast before she heard it from her friends. Everything went well, except that she was ever so mad that I hadn't told her sometime in the last 16 years. The right times just occur so infrequently in my family.

Both my sister and my niece have accompanied me down State Street in the Gay Pride Marches; I'm blessed with a supportive and loving family. The big event for the Pride weekend is a large community picnic, people come from all over the country to see and be seen. Old friendships are rekindled and new ones forged. There are races, food, music, entertainment, vendors, and beer. I was there to help with the first picnic in 1974, it was a homemade event, with a considerable amount of time spent making potato salad for hundreds, cooking, serving beer, and cleaning up the park. Over the years, it has evolved into an event where politicians shake hands and kiss babies or babes and vendors sell their wares. TV stations film it because it is so large, usually between 1,500 and 2,000 in attendance, and people can safely be who they are, or who they want to be. I quit going to these picnics in the 80s and 90s. It became increasingly difficult to overlook the fact that more and more of my friends were missing at these events. One was afraid to ask where so and so was because the most likely answer was that they were no longer with us. Magic Picnic became a sort of role call event for the Gay community, and frankly, I was seeing enough of the effects of AIDS on a daily basis, that I found that a yearly tally of the dead among us was more than I needed.

My first scare was with idiopathic thrombocytopenia purpurea (ITP). At the time, I couldn't get properly treated in Madison; I was taking about four times the recommended dose of steroids, every 6 hours! My refrigerator became my best friend. My HMO refused to call the doctors I had contacted at the Gay Men's Health Crisis Center in New York City, or the agreeing doctors at the Shanti Project in San Francisco. I made the first call to New York City and discovered that there were now 30 men presenting symptoms identical to mine, split evenly between New York and San Francisco. Cool—I was a trend setter in the Midwest. I had better get my doc to call them immediately. He wouldn't make the calls. He said that I was plainly over reacting to ITP, even though, to me, it seemed odd that I had something going on inside me that almost always occurred in middle-aged women. I left this HMO ASAP and headed over to UW to see if they would listen to me. I had my spleen removed. My T-Cell count was 900; preoperatively, my platelet count was 15,000, postoperatively it was 1,400,000, and I still lived through the surgery. I knew I was dying, so I asked my doctor to honor my wishes for a "do not resuscitate" (DNR) order, he argued, and my mom protested through tears. My dear friend Buddy just happened to be one of those 30 men; he was in New York and he decided to leave his spleen in. He died several years later. I was the first known HIV+ patient to have surgery at UW. My coworkers refused to transport me from the floor to the operating room; they went on break or took the day off. I was devastated—apparently, I was deadly in their eyes.

It had become apparent to everyone working with the HIV/AIDS community that patients needed to become very knowledgeable about treatment options. Doctors had little or no information about HIV/AIDS, and many still saw it as a big-city problem or, at the very least, a gay thing. Medical advocates went to appointments and poured over charts and scientific journals. Some of the best information was being distributed by grassroots organizations within the HIV/AIDS organizations around the world. I remember reading an article in a magazine that recommended a 50% cut in the dosage of AZT. I told my physician about it and said that I was going to cut my dose in half. I did. Six months later, my doctor told me about this article in the *Journal of the American Medical Association* (JAMA) that suggested a 50% cut in AZT doses. I listened to him thinking this all sounded very familiar to me; in fact, I had cut my dose 6 months earlier. When I pointed this out, he simply told me that I shouldn't be adjusting my dosage without consulting him first. This would not be the last time I needed to be ahead of the treating physicians, nor would it be the last time I discovered that they rarely listened to information that was being passed along to them.

Things just seemed to go from bad to worse for me. My born-again Christian cousins decided to save me before I woke up from my spleenectomy. Fortunately for me, my mother and sister managed to get into my room early and caught them huddled over me. I just don't understand why people naturally assume that I need saving. I am a deeply spiritual person. My problem is with organized religions that declare me lost from the get go. I've received hate mail from The Wisconsin Christians United because I came out in an article in the *Isthmus* (Vol. 26, No. 8/Feb 23–March 1, 2001, *www.thedailypage.com*) as a gay man with AIDS. For the most part, my encounters with organized religions have been negative, and that is being very generous on my part. I got to stare down Rev. Fred Phelps of the Westboro Baptist Church. He is famous for picketing the funeral and burial of Mathew Sheppard, the 20-something man that was crucified in Laramie, Wyoming, because the guys out West don't work and play well with those that aren't like them. Fred has a Web site devoted to hating all members of the LGBT communities and celebrating our deaths (*www.godhatesfags.com*). I grew up with a background of Fundamentalists, the Women's Temperance Union, and the KKK. All of these things seemed to be connected and I knew in my heart that I was one of those people that my background had taught me to hate. Why wouldn't I have a problem with organized religions? That doesn't mean that I need saving. My relationship with my God is my business. I've had to go through a lot, and my relationship with my God has done just fine by me. I say don't try to fix for me what isn't broken in the first place.

That night a longtime night nurse took care of me. She refused to give me pain meds, told me I was a baby, and that I had brought this all on myself. In her charting, she described me as uncooperative because I wouldn't roll without help. Jeez O Petes, I had just had major abdominal surgery, and she was withholding pain meds. I got a hold of my friends in the nursing office and asked that she not enter my room again. They told me that she was just sensitive because her son was a drug addict and gay to boot. Who cared? The next evening, a male nurse walked into my room, announced that he was a heterosexual God-fearing man, but that he'd take care of me since I had kicked D. out of my room forever. Oh boy, I could tell this was going to be a fun evening. He ignored me as much as possible and I cried.

Then there was a nasty HIV brain infection. It was thought that HIV wouldn't cross the blood-brain barrier. Boy-oh-boy, that was a wrong thought. My CNS fluid had 14 times the viral activity as was found in my blood. There was nothing to be done; my physician got me into a compassionate-use drug study with a drug called AZT. That means that the drug had not been sufficiently tested on human subjects, but it could be used as a last ditch attempt to save someone. This was an excellent source of information on the drug and its many side effects. My T Cell count was 1,200, and AZT saved my life. Unfortunately, the infection chewed up a lot of things in my brain, including my memory.

Meanwhile, back at the ranch, AIDS was wrecking havoc on the gay community. Men were dropping like flies, weekly reports from different cities showed I was losing friends in New York, Detroit, Minneapolis, Chicago, Los Angeles, San Francisco, and countless small towns that people returned to as they became increasingly ill. I had created Madison First AIDS Library at the United, set up a pamphlet distribution center at The Washington Hotel, purchased condoms by the case, and handed them out free anywhere I could. At that time it was against the law to sell them anywhere but in pharmacies, and I watched 6 members of our 7-member support group die in 2 weeks. The remaining member ran from the building never to be seen by me again. I was losing friends from all over the country. I was finding it increasingly difficult to be up for all the folks that needed me. By this time I had gotten a reputation. Dear friends and some not so dear friends were requesting my emotional support through their ordeal. Great—now I could watch my friends die up close and personal.

By this time, UW had recognized me as their leading authority on the psychosocial needs of the walking dead—that is, guys with AIDS. They even gave me a free get-out-of-parking-jail card. I was spending my 8- to 12-hour shifts on the ward, followed by hours of hand holding, and disseminating any available information to my clients at UW.

Somewhere in this timeline, I figured out that flossing your teeth was a very bad thing to do. I was flossing one night and pulled a cap off. I went to my longtime dentist to get it replaced, as he had done the original root canal and capping. I figured I had better tell him of my HIV status, which was the second big mistake of the week (the first was flossing). He pulled his hands out of my face and asked why I was there. It only made sense to me that I would come to him. That wasn't his point, which was, "Why would you throw money down a rat hole?" he was sure I would be dead before the glue dried. I told the story at work in the burn unit at UW, and the dentist at the emergency room finished the work. I didn't go back to a dentist until I found the AIDS Resource Center of Wisconsin (ARCW) HIV Dental Clinic in Milwaukee, that was 1999. My fillings were falling out like mad; they knew it was a complication of my "cocktail," a potent combination of drugs I was taking. Wisely, they have hired a very personable, knowledgeable, and brutishly handsome dentist. Going to the dentist is something I look forward to even though he has already done five root canals and caps.

Sometime in 1992, December as I recall, I noticed that my pants were fitting differently. I went to my doctor only to discover that I was in the throes of wasting syndrome, and my T-Cell count was under 200. In 3 months' time, I lost three pants sizes. Muscle mass was melting away; I didn't have any fat to lose. One of the hard things was getting pants every month that fit, so I got pants from dead men's wardrobes. We called it the Dead Guys Gap. My doctor decided to switch some of my meds around; that didn't work, and I continued losing weight. He told me once again to get my house in order, because this wasting syndrome was deadly. I went on medical leave, and I lost my health insurance, my life insurance, and my income continuation insurance due to a paper mix up. There was nowhere to turn. I couldn't afford drugs or doctors, and by God I wasn't going to spend what little time I had left throwing up after taking my new meds. I quit it all. No drugs. No doctors. No nothing. I started working at The Washington Hotel fulltime. I partied like only a dying guy can and will party. Three years later, I had gotten into a group insurance plan, and went to a doctor because I was having trouble breathing. I knew it was PCP. I had bilateral ear, nose, and pulmonary infections. She made me go back on the drugs, checking my T-Cell count, which was nearly 800. Viral loads hadn't been introduced yet.

Somewhere around this time, I started taking drug vacations. They are technically called structured treatment interruptions (STI). I had read about them in an article on *www.thebody.com*, a very informative and interactive Web site, and a magazine entitled *POZ. POZ* tells it like it is; no sidestepping issues here. According to their research, a person could benefit from an interruption in one's drug therapy. They cautioned that most doctors were unwilling to suggest this as a solution to nausea and side effects of drug therapy. I thought it sounded like a capital idea. I thought long and hard about it and decided I needed a vacation. I didn't consult doctors or friends about this because I wanted to be the responsible party if things went wrong. My first STI was for

3 months; when I had my viral load checked following the STI, there was no difference in the post- and prevacation numbers. I still didn't inform my physician for fear of another lecture on treating myself. Months later, he would mention this as a last ditch attempt to control my side effects. I've taken four STIs, and, to date, I've not had any complications from them.

You may be asking why in the world I did this. I have my reasons, but not being tied down to a very strict daily medication schedule was one of the very most important to me. People were stopping their drugs because the regimen was hard to follow, the drugs were sickening, and often they produced body-altering side effects. People were getting buffalo humps on their necks, and protease inhibitors were producing something called protease paunch—an enlargement of the belly from lipodystrophy syndrome, occurring in as many as 75% of people taking protease inhibitors. Even as your waist expands and fat accumulates around your trunk, your arms and legs are thinning and your face is wrinkling (giving you the dreaded "puppet face"). Some people have resorted to liposuction and plastic surgery to have the excess fat removed from their trunks and restored to their face and limbs, but accumulation of fat around your internal organs, high triglyceride and blood sugar levels, and reports of bone loss all make this an issue that's more than skin deep. Reports of diabetes, too, are not uncommon.

Then there is the issue of compliance. Doctors were befuddled as to why patients couldn't just take their drugs when they were supposed to. At an international conference on AIDS, doctors were given sugar pills, and instructed to take them according to various treatment regiments that their patients were on. This was going to be a weeklong experiment. Some medications require that the patient is nothing by mouth (npo) 2 hours before ingesting the medication and 1 hour after ingesting it. These medications were taken three or four times a day. After the week long trial was over, it was discovered that there was over 90% noncompliance from the physicians. This was one week, we are on these drugs for the rest of our lives, and most people required to take these drugs are not physicians and have very little knowledge of the adverse effects of missing a dose. No wonder there was noncompliance among the HIV/AIDS community, the people prescribing them couldn't even adhere to the regimens for a week.

In July of 1990, one of my dearest friends died of lymphoma of the brain. It was a particularly difficult death for me to experience. I met him when I was 17 and was illegally in his bar, but we hit it off. An older cousin of mine had found this bar he thought that I would like. I would turn 18 in 2 months, so I was almost legal. That was 1972; we spent 18 years really caring about one another. We were best buds. Toward the end, I had to lie in his bed with him; he was too weak to get up. Rodney Scheel, the owner of the Washington Hotel, the Back Door, and a driving force in Madison's Gay and Lesbian Community died in July 1990. I didn't know how to deal with this; the guy I always could turn to was dead. So, I put together a production company and raised money to help open the Rodney Scheel House.

My friend Mark and I couldn't think of a good name for the production company, so we simply asked what people thought of when they saw us—we who were always together doing something, and usually something naughty. Our friend Dennis gave us the perfect name: Potential Mayhem. We had three benefit events, had a whole lot of fun, and realized that people were willing to give us money like mad if we'd only get up on stage and make fools of ourselves. The last benefit we organized was a bit much; I ended up in the hospital with fingers the size of brats. They were infected with something nasty and had to be hung from IV poles; the doctors were mentioning the possibility of amputation because of septic knuckles. So, I got a pass and spent the night at the Great Hall in the Memorial Union surrounded by drag queens and kings, my family, and my friends and wishing once again that I would wake up from this nightmare.

In October of 1993, at the tender age of 38, I had to have my appendix removed. Apparently, HIV stuff can accumulate in your appendix. And I thought that I had everything removed that I could; besides, appendix were removed in children, not adults. I was wrong. While I was hospitalized, I discovered that I had no insurance coverage. After leaving, I was bankrupt; I had medical bills coming due, a mortgagee I couldn't pay, and a pending lawsuit nearing $100,000 because my dog injured someone else's dog, eventually leading to that dog's demise. I filed for bankruptcy, lost my house, and ended up living in the Rodney Scheel House. If you wait, it all comes full circle.

Last month, I went to have a fatty tumor removed from under my right eye. This month I go in for the Mohs procedure to remove basal cell carcinomas from my face. Medications from Ambein to Zoloft, with plenty of common antibiotics, antidepressants, and antiinflammatories in between, can make you more sensitive to the sun. In addition, sun may make you vulnerable to recurrences of herpes, rosacea, and other problems. AIDS-pioneer Marcus Conant, an assistant dermatologist at the University; of California at Los Angeles, suggests that long exposure to the sun may boost levels of HIV itself in positive men with low CD4-cell counts. Among the medications and herbs causing photosensitivity are sulfa or tetracycline-based antibiotics, sleeping pills, antidepressants, antianxiety medications, and all tricyclic antidepressants, Saint John's wort, antiinflammatories, and antihistamines. I still get fairly nauseated on a regular basis from my meds and fairly disgusted at the lack of definitive answers to questions about side effects and their treatment.

I am still volunteering at MASN, and I do speaking engagements. I speak to educate. Education is a key part to understanding. Bigotry and hate are usually the products of ignorance, and by speaking to the graduating class of nursing students, I hope to make vague concepts a reality. I remember my first days in nursing. I was afraid of just about everything and every patient around me. One thing I have learned through my personal experience with a chronic disease is that there isn't a thing that you can ask or say to me that hasn't run through my head. I think about death, I think about being sick and disabled. I sometimes think about being hooked up to machines keeping me alive and wonder what kind of life that would be for me and for the people that love me. I get angry when a medical professional announces that they know what I'm going through. That's impossible, how can any of you know what it is like for me to live through this? None of you know the devastating affects the AIDS pandemic has had on my life. I wonder how many of you have lost hundreds of friends and watched countless young people die from a disease that your government and president wouldn't even name? Do you understand the depth of my anger and hurt? Do you understand the shame and guilt that religious groups can cast upon you for loving whom you love or being who you are? It runs deep. Do you understand that after listening to medical professionals joke about patients' sexual orientation, there is a certain basic mistrust that I carry with me just as surely as I carry my PJ's and toothbrush?

It is not any one's place to judge me, the patient, for living my life the best I can. We are all born, and we live life the best we can and then die. I happened to become infected with a virus—nothing but a virus. That's what I want to be treated for. I don't care what your views are on most subjects, particularly ones that have no bearing on my medical well being. I want my basic emotional and medical needs addressed; I don't want you to try to fix anything else you perceive as being wrong with me.

Twice a year, I come in and discuss things with you that most people try to keep private. Why? There are an infinite number of answers to this question, but I have only a few reasons to make myself this vulnerable. I come in and lay my soul bare so that you can safely ask questions that are knocking about your brain. I come in because right now, there is an alarming trend among people to put AIDS/HIV on the back burner because there are drugs. AIDS/HIV still kills. AIDS/HIV still makes live incredibly difficult and still makes one sick as hell. There is no cure. I hear how excited people are about a possible vaccine. I'm not very excited; a vaccine won't do a thing for me or the millions of people like me that have AIDS/HIV. I speak to you because no matter how much information there is about the odds and chances of getting AIDS/HIV, when you get it, the odds and chances are meaningless. I speak to you because if I had a genetic disease, I might seem more acceptable to you. I speak to you because someday, you could be taking care of me, and, hopefully, you will remember me and give me that extra care that may just get me over the hump. I also speak to you because I know your instructor would hunt me down if I didn't. I also speak to you because, after almost 20 years, AIDS/HIV has taken its toll on me, and I don't have the energy to do the big-ticket items. Been there, done that, didn't even get a T shirt. I speak to you because I can.

I also speak for selfish reasons. Speaking makes me feel like I am doing something in the war on AIDS/HIV. It makes me feel good. I also get taken to lunch if I do a good job; at the very least, I get coffee and snacks. I speak for my own well-being. If I do good things, good things will happen to me; I think it is called *karma*. I tell you my stories so that you can put a face on this most evil disease.

I write this to remember. I write this to help you understand. I never want to forget those I've lost. I want compassion for those that suffer. I tell stories from the past so that history doesn't repeat itself. I don't know why I've lived and why so many others with my condition have died.

One day, I expect the other shoe to drop. I keep envisioning the scene from *A Longtime Companion*. Everybody that has died of AIDS in the movie has gathered down at the beach for a big old tea dance. The remaining characters stumble onto this most joyous celebration. A song plays—I think it is "The Rigor Mortis Café," you see all the folks meeting again, dancing again, loving again. I hope something like that happens; I want to party with my friends again.

John's Story

I met Adrian sometime in the mid 70s, either late 1976 or very early 1977 more likely. He was standing in the dark space along the back wall of the bar. Adrian and I formed enough of a bond to become brothers, in a way. After the first month brought the realization to him that I wasn't going to be the boyfriend he was looking for, he spent the next 6 months staring at the blank wall in my apartment. He'd make it off to work sometimes, and that was about it. I think he wondered what it was he'd got himself into, and, was anyone going to be there at the other end? I had myself to take care of. We were headed in different directions on our coping paths, but I didn't ever consider throwing him out. He could stay until he felt he had his feet on the ground, and then we'd go from there. By the time that was over, we were pretty attached. I took care of him as best I could.

One has to imagine growing up gay in the 50s and 60s in rural Wisconsin. Adrian and I were both farm boys. Our experiences had been similar, but there were critical differences. We were from different faith communities. Mine was a strict Irish/German Catholic tradition. My mother's family were all school teachers, and my father's family were all musicians or great sportsmen. My grandfather and great grandfather had been choir directors, as was my father, so we had a family position to maintain in the community. There was no financial gain to be had for this position, mind you. Our situation was purely one of humility and poverty, but nonetheless "We can always do better" was the unofficial family slogan.

Adrian and I were stretching the links of the bonds we had formed toward breaking. Everything being equal, had HIV not come along, they might have broken. In my frustration and with my breaks from work I would check out for a week at a time. I constructed my schedule so that I could work 7 days in a row and then take a week off. At work, I was dedicated to being a role-model nurse/health caretaker (role playing a life). On days off, I went about my isolation with reading and art. I made occasional contacts with the outside world and maintained a few key connections. I needed the time to check out. Adrian says I still spend too much time in my head.

My personal situation was very tenuous. It took a lot of emotional energy for me to hold myself together. There are many things about my past that I do not reveal to most people but which have acted on me in a very base way. When I was 8, I began a sexual relationship with my dentist—not so willingly and not really with my permission—which lasted until I was 16. I was frightened out of my head, but he paid me money for it afterward and warned me not to tell anyone. I very shortly felt complicit in the acts. I used the money to buy records at the store around the corner from the dentist's second-floor office. Over the course of 8 years, I had most of the teeth in my mouth worked on during appointments scheduled just before lunch—or as the last of the afternoon appointments, so that the dentist's wife would go home while he finished up with me. Only long after did I wonder if I actually needed all of that dental work. At the time, I recall Dad commenting on how the dentist was giving us a break on the dental bills. I would eventually come to think of myself as a prostitute.

I've been in conversations with other gay men who initiated relationships with older boys or young men when they were as young as 14 and found the experience liberating. Their experiences were significantly different from mine. It is one thing to seek out the contact. It's another to have it begin at such an early age prior to adolescence's even beginning. There is a naturalness in a teenager seeking sexual exploration. In no way am I condoning inappropriate contact between adults and teenagers. My point is that there is a difference between seeking and exploration as a youth and being preyed upon by an adult. I feel that my ability to grow into my own sexuality was stolen.

After this dentist left our town to retire in Florida (I was 16), I put the experiences with him out of my mind. I recall the relief, though, that things were looking up. Soon, I would move away and go on to college. This had long been my target and pathway away from this unhappy existence. I loved the land and exploring the spaces around the farm, local creeks, woods, springs, and rivers, but the culture was stifling. My parents and extended family and similar local families insisted on excellence in behavior and performance, but there was another strong tradition of not succeeding at school. This outlook viewed education as a big waste of time. I wanted none of this tradition.

My family and the local culture was one where sex was never discussed except in the form of a little seldom seen church pamphlet, which I've kept somewhere. Loving touch between my parents was never seen in the house. I think they viewed it as immoral and a bad example. I don't know, maybe they were ashamed or afraid. Sex was not for enjoyment, only for producing children, so affection might have been viewed as risky behavior. Dating was discouraged.

I was in a university chemistry class when the smell of ether in a lab demonstration reawakened an incident from when I was 11 or so. The memory is of waking up on my stomach on the dentist's office couch with his weight heavy on my back. As soon as he realized I was awake, he stuffed an ether rag to my nose and I passed out again. That smell of ether will always be associated deep inside my brain somewhere with this experience and memory. Not something I choose to recall. The recall is engraved into my brain chemistry. I walked back to school that day quite dazed—and probably hung over from the large ether dose—wondering just what had happened to me and what it meant, and feeling something wet drip down my bottom side.

I retreated to the university library as soon as I could and began my research. The only literature on homosexuality was in the form of delinquency and prison reports. Sexual abusers were often themselves abused and so the theory of this cycle of abuse was the explanation for this type of delinquency. There was no literature available on any sense of a normalcy in gay evolution. The American Psychiatric Association (APA) was not to take homosexuality off of the disease lists until after 1973 or so. I had no doubt I was attracted to men. For me this had been a long-term given. I resented not having the ability to develop a natural sense of my own sexuality. This is one of the things of which I had been robbed.

In order to function on a day-to-day basis during stress, I needed to follow a strict structure and regimen, then secure a space where I could feel safe afterward and decompress. This was the nature and intent of my isolation—the seeking of a safe environment. I so wanted it to be different, but these retreats created safe situations where I could relax and begin to think about how to deal with the rest of the world and my life. Stressful circumstances can present themselves at somewhat predictable times in a work situation. I could use this experience and test and practice my coping skills by the controlled stress of the work situation where there were others to rely on. I didn't reveal to anyone my method, but it provided me a controlled environment for positive growth.

Adrian and I were driving near home one night when the news was reported on "All Things Considered" that a number of cases of a rare form of cancer was being reported among a number of gay men in New York City and San Francisco, and they didn't know what the cause or relationship was between the cases. Adrian and I looked at one another and drove on in silence, both aware that this could be infectious and that we had links with both communities. My interpretation at hearing the news was that we individually were at risk. I think Adrian's response was more that our community was at risk.

I said we needed to become the healthiest people on the planet to prepare to handle what might be coming on. I'd already been headed down this road. It was a reconnection with the earlier beliefs and priorities of my youth. I was a nature boy, Adrian was social. I quit going to bars. I decided I didn't want to live in a smoky house and Adrian's smoking was a problem for me. I would get back into growing my garden and harvesting from the wild, exercising, eating well, and preparing myself to live a good life. I'd studied self-actualization and wanted to become self-actualized. I would implement a plan to attempt to achieve that goal.

Adrian and I spoke about how the individual going through this would be treated. We both realized we would have to take care of each other because no one else was going to care enough to do it. Adrian could shine in a crisis. He acted out of his heart. We had no notion of how this would come to affect us personally. Shortly, Adrian came home from work with his first story of a gay man admitted and put in strict isolation. All the medical staff were afraid to go in to see the man. The minimal care that could be given was done. People talked with disgust about the life style of these men and how they deserved what they were getting, but "why did they have to assign us the chore of taking care of them?"

My focus was on how I was going to respond to this environmental change around me. My first act was to come out to my mother. If I had this thing, I needed to warn my mother, and, subsequently the rest of my family, ahead of time so that when the time came for me to die, there would not be wasted time and energy spent trying to tell them I was gay, sick, and dying. I thought if I could prepare the groundwork ahead of time, there would be an opportunity for all of us in the family to prepare ourselves to the best of our abilities. I thought being honest and up front was my best option. What did I have to lose? At worst, I could be wrong and get my being gay off of my chest once and for all.

There was no way to know for sure if I would have this thing until something happened. I was admitting something might happen. I wanted them to be over the phase of shock. I wanted them to be able to help me if I needed it. I didn't want to spend my last days fighting with them over who I was. After I told her, Mum said she'd always suspected I was gay. I said I was doing all I could to live as healthy a life as I could and I tried to help other people as best as I was able and as they'd taught me. She said that was all anyone could do and thanked me for being honest and up front with her.

I also told her about the sexual actions of our family and town's dentist and would learn some shocking information over the next month or so as I continued my conversations with my mother. It turns out that this dentist had tried to attack my uncle 40 years earlier and he had been strong enough to say "no." What was wrong with me that I wasn't? I knew I wasn't the only individual who'd been used by this man, but I had no idea it had been going on for this long and nothing had ever been done about it. I was so angry. How many other lives had been affected? Was so and so's suicide related? Other circumstances? I knew there had been some common knowledge about these practices. There were jokes about this dentist in our town. I thought people maybe knew that I was involved with him and so were teasing me. This could have been the case, as the dentist had mentioned a name or two of other town boys and asked if I ever played with them sexually. He likely asked these others if they'd played with me, too. True enough, my family didn't hang around with the sort of people who joked like that, so it's possible they never heard anything about these circumstances before I spoke up. My reward was being blamed for the abuse.

Then Adrian told me he was bruising easily and all over the place and what was he going to do about it. He'd called around and knew that this was part of what some clinics were seeing. They thought it might be a milder form of what was going around or just the first stage. No one knew. My new partner (a physician) and I went to see Adrian together at his house to find out what support we could offer. He had an upcoming doctor's appointment. At this point in my life, I was still in no shape to deal with someone else's struggle on the front line. My partner went along to Adrian's appointment instead of me, but I promised before my new partner and to Adrian that I would be there to take care of Adrian, whatever happened. This was our extended family. We would continue to rally for each other.

This was a very dark period for all of us. Adrian could expect a few months at best. I'd stopped planning for any future, too, ever since hearing the news of this gay plague. I had to be prepared for what might be lurking around the next corner. I had to prepare myself, be ever vigilant. I had to prepare myself to cope with the difficult task of terminal care for this person whose life I'd affected and who had affected mine deeply. Now I was not only going to lose him, but I was going to take care of him while he left. I would be up to it. This was all part of my commitment to Adrian. I was lucky to have a new partner who understood the depth of this relationship and did not perceive it as a threat. I also needed to be grounded somewhere else. My new partner would need to play that role for me.

Adrian and I began a series of "last trips." A strong part of our bond had formed over camping trips to canyon lands where we would hike and read. Adrian was deeply into reading Anasazi petroglyphs and pictographs and had identified a significant site where he wanted his ashes spread. I was deeper and deeper into my exploration of art, culture, and techniques for living and understanding a life—my own— and comparing and melding this with all the life I came across. Connections with past and future life were more rewarding than much of the present life we came across, so the archeology and the anthropologic focus was shared between us. These trips continued, though I was now in a new relationship. These were my terms and my priorities. There were not always acceptable to the others in my life, and that was something we had to suffer through. It was understandable.

Adrian kept living, and living, throughout the 80s and into the 90s. He was losing friends and acquaintances and individuals whom he was caring for. This constant loss was almost worse. Survivor's guilt is real, and his tendency was to revert back to parties, alcohol, and drugs to forget about what was going on and pass the times with these friends, who could help him forget. My losses were distanced. I knew of some of the people who would die over the years, but only as acquaintances. No one that I was close to or had remained in touch with, with several key exceptions (my first partner was one), died. I was off in isolation land, as usual, and working more and more.

In July 1992, I got a needle-stick injury while at work taking care of a young individual with multisystem organ failure, unknown etiology. It appeared to be some fulminant process, so the needle-stick risk was heightened. If I was now HIV negative, the only risk to me of being tested was to find that out and make sure that I could establish that condition in case I came down with something new as a result of this injury, and so I debated only a short time. After discussions with my partner, I got tested the next day at work and within a few days was called into the employee health office for a visit with the head of infectious diseases, who informed me that I had advanced HIV disease. I was given what must have been the usual time span for predictive survival: 6 to (at best) 18 months. The advice was that I had better get my papers in order.

Even though I'd lived with this cloud over my head for years, I'd gotten used to it and had begun to believe that I'd escaped—that I was one of the lucky ones of my generation. Now the truth was shaking me into another reality. I remained as calm as I could outwardly and continued to work. I didn't reveal my diagnosis to my work mates. I took it as my mission to continue to do my work responsibly as long as I had to and adapt to the changes with the help of the few friends I did tell. The first of these friends was Adrian. My partner came with me to tell him. This was one of the hardest things to do because I had promised to take care of Adrian, and now I was presenting a scenario where I, too, might soon get sick and die, and Adrian would have to sit through this and watch, and be a survivor.

By this time, there had been viral tests available for some time, but I was not sexually active outside of my relationship, and my partner and I were careful and safe. He remained HIV negative throughout. My partner had assured me that I couldn't be positive and that, anyway, there was no reason to be tested as there was no real treatment available. The drugs that were being used (AZT & DDC is what I recall starting on) were not great at doing much other than slowing down the process a little, and then resistance took over. The main reason for not being tested was the great risk of losing all my insurance coverage the moment this was on my record. There were minimal or no protections against such actions, and even if I was successful at meeting all of my obligations toward insurance payments, there seemed to be filing measures that intervened negatively on the part of other individuals to cause them to lose coverage. My partner, after finishing residency, and I had managed to stay close to Madison, where I could continue to work without having to change job locations and risk any insurance check or change in the process.

I had new drugs to get used to, new doctors to see, a frequent regimen of lab work followed by the anxiety of the results, work, and the added pressure of trying to figure out how to tell my family about this diagnosis. I didn't have much time. I'd been very cautious for years about hand washing and cleanliness both at work and at home or with family. My sister-in-law, a nurse, recognized a change in my behavior about 3 months into this and guessed the answer. You can't really hide major changes from the people who know you best. She asked if I'd told my mother, and I said I'd not because I was trying to work up to it—mostly postponing, I suppose. It was too emotional for me to talk about yet, and I felt I needed to get to a point where I was sufficiently in control that I could respond to and be prepared to offer comfort.

What response could I expect? I didn't think about that directly, and it was not what held me back. I was worried about how my mother would respond and what kind of support system she would have for her grief. How could I cushion the blow? I wanted to set up a support system ahead of time so that she would have someone to talk with about this news to help her process it. I thought if I prepared my two sisters, who lived nearby and worked in hospital settings, then she would have their support. How was I to do that? I would first need to tell my sisters, allow them time to get over it and used to it, and be in a position to be available (when they were no longer in shock over the diagnosis) to be able to help Mum and Dad through the news. My sister-in-law said I should not wait, and we set up a visit shortly thereafter when I would tell Mum and Dad with my sister-in-law present to give support.

It wasn't easy and didn't go well. I didn't go to the farm; Mum and Dad came to my house instead. They were uncomfortable in my house because of my partnership relationship. I grew up Catholic, and they'd always said they could love the sinner but not the sin. They recognized and admitted that I was a caring and highly spiritual person, but there was dissonance in that I refused to deny or be shamed by my sexuality and insisted on recognition for my partnership. Mum had said in the past that she thought it was important that I have someone to live with, too, and my partner was a very good man. I'd helped many family members in little ways, and my partner had helped intervene. I had spent time with my brother and his family during his bone-marrow transplant, which was successful in itself, but was not successful in the end, as the scar tissue from the pretreatment took over. I helped to determine it was time to let him go. (I'd worked with bone-marrow transplants. I was the only one in the family with this level of expertise. They relied on me.)

Now my diagnosis placed me—in the eyes of much of society—in that lowest category of human, namely, those who deserved to get HIV because of their chosen lifestyle, and this was clear evidence of God's retribution and punishment for my behavior. I would have to sleep in the bed I made. All my efforts at self-improvement were set to go down the drain by this mark of HIV+. All my good deeds and efforts were to be overruled by this mark. This was the view of much of society, then, only 11 years ago. How much has that changed? It has, but that's another story.

After I told my parents about my diagnosis, things were difficult. My focus was on issues of paperwork and coping. I had to figure out what was important to keep, what was important to try and complete, and what I could afford to whittle away or let go. I worked for another year, until I found myself so tired and fatigued at work that I was afraid my performance was putting my patients and fellow staff at risk. I'd used up all of my sick time. I took a two-week vacation and ended up sleeping through most of it. I came back from this vacation having discussed with my partner that I felt I could not continue to work—that I was unsafe and that it was unfair to others. However, I didn't want to have to say goodbye to the staff I worked with. This was cowardly of me, but it was the course I chose.

I went to the nursing department in the hospital—told them what was going on and how I didn't feel I could go on with work anymore. I cried at having to give up my connections and my profession in this way. They arranged to schedule my departure notice as vacation time and would handle the contact and scheduling issues my absence would create. As a nurse with many years of practice experience, I knew how much we depended on each other to carry our load, how difficult it could be when someone took unexpected time off, and knew that most of us were prepared for just this sort of event. Unexpected and unexplained things happen. I trusted the people I worked with, whom I loved to work with, would come to understand. A unit forms a bond unique to the unit and it's members. There's a family of support in nursing care. We individually depend on each other to help us be there for our patients in their difficult moments. Care could be fairly routine, but routine was as likely to be disrupted by some unexpected crisis at any time. We individually coped as a group in many ways in my unit. I was aware of my responsibility in this matter. It was no small thing for me to leave.

At home, I was paralyzed. I had insurance and disability papers of all sorts to deal with. Never my strength, paper work now became my life and drove me nearly insane. My thinking was not very clear as is. I was very fatigued and a bit depressed, to say the least. Depression had always been an issue I'd had to deal with. Oh, it probably ran in my family, no doubt, and my own past had contributed its degree of reasons to feel down about myself. This was a prime time to sink into it all (it was fall, going into winter).

My social contacts had almost all been work related, and now these were gone. The community where I lived, though 50 minutes from work, was a community in which I had no connections other than my partner. He worked long, difficult hours, had his own worries about how he was going to cope with my difficulties and our life together until I died, and then what was he to do? He and I already had our papers in order, but there's so much more that needs to be prepared for that one can't easily get a handle on. Actual and anticipatory grief were big factors affecting him.

By 1996, I was down to 20 and then 10 T-cells for 6–8 months. My mother was experiencing some of the earlier signs of the Alzheimer's disease, which seemed to run in her family line. I had guilt over the fact that the stress from my diagnosis revelation back in 1992 had begun this slide downhill into a more distanced and scattered response. While I understand that I ought not blame myself for what was happening to her, I knew the toll stress could take on an individual and how it could precipitate other illness. Mother and I had always been very close. I was a difficult child (an understatement). The family always called me the black sheep of the family. I was always misbehaving, getting into everything, and so on. As a child, I was classically hyperactive, with attention deficit disorder prior to that diagnosic process gaining favor. Mum spent a lot of extra time with me, especially on Sundays, when she would take me to church early with her, and then I could spend the morning at home playing on my own and helping to set the dinner table while the rest of my 10 siblings were off to church with Dad.

How long could this life go on? I had already completed most of the narrowing of my interests to a few—my art, my family contact, and some light travel. My partner was preparing for me to die, as was I. I tried to arrange my funeral plans. I wanted to be cremated—not acceptable to my local parish. I could try and specify that in my will, but once I was dead, it was meaningless, because next of kin would need to sign for the disposal of my body, and my partner, for all the paper work we'd done, could not be considered next of kin. I called the local priest and asked about the rules on cremation and learned that it was permissible in cases, but why would I want to deny my family the opportunity for a Catholic burial? I moved to ask a more sympathetic sibling to assume responsibility for signing my death certificate placing in them the faith that they would approve my partners and my wishes for cremation. This was to be my last act, I expected.

Then, miraculously, protease inhibitors came on the market. I took the first one available and got wildly sick. It was Retonivir. We commonly referred to it as "retchtonivir" because of the nausea it caused. It gave my mouth a heavy metallic taste. By the end of one week of dosing, I was retching so badly I needed to be admitted into the hospital (my first hospitalization for AIDS-related issues). I'd been hospitalized several times previously—briefly—for atrial fib, unknown etiology (most likely stress related).

I figured this was my luck, and the protease inhibitors weren't going to be working for me, so I reset my mind to accept the coming end of my life. My physician waited for me to recover from this spell and then persuaded me to try a second protease inhibitor, which I did. This was Crixivan. I responded with no problem. Within a few months, my T-cells were moving into a range in which I was presented with an option to try and get into a new clinical trial using Interleukin II (IL2) as an immune stimulator. We just needed to get my T-cell count up to 200 for me to qualify. That seemed like an incredibly high watermark for me. I was told that T-cell counts were usually highest early in the morning, so that's when I got my testing done, and my count was exactly 200, so I was in the study.

The idea with IL2 was that it could possibly stimulate stem cell production of T-cells by mimicking viral flu-like symptoms. The effect would last for a while, and then, on a regularly scheduled basis, I'd dose over again. This was a stage 3-trial, which meant it had been through several steps and proved to be a reasonable treatment option. The next step would be general/limited approval for use. I was getting an early shot at the protocol.

The dosing involved subcutaneous shots in the abdomen twice a day for 7 days. If the fever, shaking chills, and nausea that resulted were too severe, doses near the end could be skipped. The effect was cumulative. Each dose created a stronger response that built on the previous. Eventually, I could predict when the shaking chills and fevers and nausea would occur and when it would seem reasonable to get up and move around a little. I can't adequately express how severe the symptoms of the fever and chills would get. Each site of injection would gradually swell up, turn red and tender, and then gradually subside. This was week 1 of the process. Week 2 was recovery week. I was still fairly sick—more wiped out than anything, and limited more by the painful injection sites as they diminished than continued fevers, though they persisted somewhat as well. Week 3–7, I would sometimes feel quite a bit better. I'd feel an energy peak, but then a gradual decline in energy as I slid back toward my dosing time at the 8th week, when the process started all over again. Not only did the dosing effects increase in degree with each individual dose, but, over time, the effects from subsequent dosing periods built upon each other. Not all of these effects were beneficial. One of the nonbeneficial effects was that it began to appear that dosing magnified some preexisting psychiatric effects in some individuals.

With me, this was depression. Week 2 became an immensely and deepening tunnel of depression I would fall into. Initially, it was just crying at anything—even commercials. Eventually, before they finally stopped my treatments, it had become a huge vacuum I fell into and couldn't begin to find my way out of. There were conflicting events going on. My T-cells had recovered to nearly 500 and remained steady. My base energy had increased, but I still retained significant fatigue and continued to sleep for extended periods (12–16 hours a day). More important, my outlook had changed. Protease Inhibitors were being talked about as a possible miracle cure for people with AIDS. Suddenly, I was no longer looking death in the face. I might still have a life ahead of me. I had hope. For the first time in years, I felt that I could begin to plan for a future, tentative as it might be. I as a model patient, immensely compliant with my medication regimen, which is key to reducing resistance issues, and I remained physically isolated from new or risky infection. Much more than this, I had the knowledge and support to do my research and proceed with my plan to be as healthy as I could possibly be.

My home situation changed, too. I was no longer willing to compromise with my partner on certain relationship issues. He had to make significant shifts in his thinking as well. He'd been preparing himself for taking care of me as I died, and now I wasn't going to die—at least not as soon as we'd expected. That meant we needed to renegotiate how we lived together. I had new demands. While ill, I had narrowed my interests and focus down to the few things of real import to me. I wasn't going to *expand* that list now, but I would take every chance I could to *express* that list. I began to sing in a gay choral group, and I got involved in community theater. This for me, as someone who would earlier have described himself as morbidly shy, was amazing. I was breaking out and taking on new challenges. This was my last chance to flower, I thought. I had better step into it. No wasting time now.

I think it is not uncommon, when someone receives such a reprieve on what has appeared to be a certain death sentence, to come out of that with some risk to his immediate relationship structures. I had prepared myself to move out twice before I met someone else who tipped the emotional scales. I told my partner I'd met someone else before anything more happened, and it was some time before anything more would happen, but the cast was set and I was to end the relationship as we knew it.

The subsequent events I feel less comfortable discussing. Let's just admit it didn't work out. I knew it was not a likely success scenario to leave one relationship for someone else, but I did, and almost as suddenly as I had, that new relationship began to fail.

I avoided focusing on failure—but only after a long recovery time— and I regained stability, avoided several old traps, got into long-term counseling, and continued my outreach work in areas of personal interest (landscape design and restoration, community involvement and participation, and my art). My energy levels are still at risk. I can push myself for a short time beyond my routine limits, but if I fail to get sufficient rest, I begin to get sick quite quickly. I must be constantly aware of the stress level that I am exposed to and evaluate my level of involvement based on what I believe I can tolerate. I continue to hide my diagnosis from some individuals. I don't think of it as hiding, really, it's just not what I want to be first on my list of topics for discussion. If I get to know someone better over time, and the opportunity presents itself, I will tell the individual or couple that I have AIDS and outline my limitations. I try not to make a big deal about it, however. That's a choice I make. I don't want my life driven by some infection I have and the medications I need to take. I'm more than that. I accept the condition as is. What are my choices?

Adrian and I again live together, and it's a good relationship—most of the time. Truth be told, he can drive me crazy. He tells me I live too much in my head. I still spend lots of time worrying about things that haven't happened yet, but I'm learning. When I'm lost in thought, I don't like to be disturbed. That's my hermit phase. I think he needs more social outlets, and he surely ain't gonna get 'em from me! So, instead, he got himself a kitty!

It's not the relationship you might imagine. I don't think anyone would call us lovers. We're not really physical beyond an occasional hug. I find I'm not interested in the partnership thing. Aw, sometimes I long for that old romance, but no one of interest presents themselves. I've gotten pretty picky and weigh the risk to me of involvement that might lead to failure. I wonder at asking someone to get to know me to the degree that would actually prove satisfying. I'm so much less willing to reveal myself or to compromise. It's a lot to ask of someone else, isn't it?

My physician ex remains both Adrian's and my medical power of attorney and health advocate, and we all get along very well. I guess we make a different sort of family. I'm glad we can find a means of remaining involved in each others lives. I recall friends/ acquaintances from nursing school with whom I was close but who did not know my whole story because I had not the guts to come out to them. These relationships leave holes, significant times that I can not draw on because the shared memories are triggered more by the remembrance of the individual—their voice, their face—than by anything less tangible. So these empty spaces remain. That is life. It's less important that it happens than that one becomes aware of it, and of how and why it happens, and is then able to make decisions and changes so that these empty spaces will form with less frequency with those whom we consider important in our lives.

So why do Adrian and I agree to speak out? What do we have to offer that is so special? I don't know that we have anything unique beyond ourselves to offer. There are many other unique stories that can be told. We have grown together and reached significant points of commonality in our process, which has placed us in the unique position of being available to speak out; this is a matter of circumstances, chance, and choice.

I think it is important to realize when you are dealing with an individual with an illness that they are so much more than their illness. Individuals carry their past and present on their shoulders. How broadly can I make my statements and have them be applicable? As a gay man, I will tell you that if you come to me making assumptions, I will detect it. I would ask you to have compassion for the individual and recognize that there may be many factors affecting the individual. When I hear about the sex scandal involving priests in the Catholic Church, I am taken back to my own experiences with child sexual abuse. I may cry all over again, though usually it is not the case that my emotions are so much on the surface. I exercise more control over my emotions than you can ever imagine—unless you have had a similar experience.

Recently, I was at a dinner party where someone made the joke that I was not into 10-year-olds. He was referring to 10-year aged cheese, but it was a turn of phrase that was enough to send me, given the condition I was in, off the edge. No, I'm not into 10-year-olds. In fact,

I *was* that 10-year-old, and I don't think it's something to be joked about. When something like that happens out of the blue, it affects you in strange ways. It's unexpected. The trigger's been pulled, and now a cascade of emotions and responses begin. When I was younger and inexperienced, I was less likely to understand what the triggers were or when they'd been pulled, but the cascade would occur regardless. One won't always recognize when their particular trigger has been pulled. The responses become automatic. It's flight or fight.

I ask you to beware of judging others. There are behaviors that are clearly unacceptable, and these limits need to be set for all individuals, but these limits will seldom be the issue you need to deal with. More likely, you will be confronted with some individual who stimulates a gut response from you. In our case, you may share the gut response that gay people are sinners, or that they choose their identity rather than being born that way. You may have a deep-seated belief that we are unclean or are untouchables and undeserving of care and concern. You may have grown up around these attitudes, believe yourself to be immune to them, and still find they have affected your interaction with the individual in question. Something about the way someone is dressed or cares for themselves may influence you to judge them in a particular manner. It's not that we don't all do those automatically, but if you are unaware of it and act out of this blindness, you are not caring for an individual. Instead, you are caring for a preconception—*your* preconception.

When Adrian and I started speaking together regarding living with HIV in a chronic-health-issues class, I didn't realize I would end up talking about much more than AIDS. Who I am and how I respond to stress and crisis is a complex result of what I've experienced and learned over many years—over my entire life. Which chronic condition is more important? Post-traumatic stress disorder as a result of child sexual abuse? Attention deficit hyperactivity disorder? Chronic depression? AIDS? Can I separate them?

Few of your HIV clients will have the medical experience, resource advocates, and skills the two of us share. Many of them will enter any system with a significant degree of mistrust. Gay people have grown to expect negative judgment. People who are not of the privileged class (in terms of color, education, income, status) may be on guard in anticipation of mistreatment

Live my life better than I did, and then you may have the right to criticize or judge me. Cripple me by placing me in a society that starts out by demeaning me as a detestable aberrancy, screw me over literally and culturally, isolate me within a shaming and blaming belief system, and expect me to grow up into a contributing member of society? You've got to be kidding! If there's any shaming to be done here, it's of the dominant culture that allowed dentists like mine to practice in towns like mine for over 40 years and did nothing about it but blame the child for letting the abuse happen. These priest abuse cases—every time I hear about one, it brings all of my experience back to me. You never get over a shaming culture. The only choice the individual has is to work to change it so that it will be better for the next generations. That's your only hope for retribution.

I made a pledge when I decided I needed to forgive my dentist and let the anger go or else it would kill me. My pledge was that I would not remain silent. This is the meaning of "Silence = Death!" This is my gay agenda. My anger swells even now as I write these sentences because the abuse in this culture continues, and it is wrong. It must stop. Not just the obvious abuse, which we all can agree now, finally, is unacceptable, but the way this culture still abuses the individual by cultural precepts that predetermine that some individuals are more worthy of all of life's experiences than are a certain minority of individuals. I'm speaking of the right to fall in love freely with someone and choose to be married and have the state recognize that relationship as an authentic expression for those individuals. Keep your church and belief system out of my life and my government. My people need that level of support from the majority culture to be whole and complete. Anyone of us may choose not to follow the path of marriage. All paths must be open to all people to choose, not arbitrarily closed off by the whims of the majority who think they know better. Let God be my judge.

My anger is focused and strong. It will not die with me. It will infect the culture from every angle. You can turn against it and fight or acquiesce and love. It's your choice. Above all else, love.

This is why we speak out. We must choose to live together with respect. Respect that is demanded without reward ends in the crucifixion of the individual who asks for respect (e.g., the murder of Matthew Shephard, as the most extreme case). We must be heard, and the majority culture must choose to give respect. It will only happen when the majority culture chooses to do what is right by all peoples and lets go of its selfish need to dominate in matters of the spirit. Do you wonder why any downgraded people turn toward nihilistic experience? Can you understand how the projected view of the group on the individual, over time, becomes internalized? The isolated individual no longer needs the larger culture to degrade them. The culturally degraded individual becomes very good at degrading himself or herself to survive, and some of these individuals form clusters of self help and support groups that are out of sight most of the time from the majority. Within these ghettos of culture, there is free expression and growth of different life experiences. What makes the gay experience unique within this cultural concept is that the gay individual springs from all sets of the broader culture and is nurtured by that broader culture until such a time as like-minded individuals are found. Without this broader cultural support, too many individuals are lost along the way.

Index

Acquired immunodeficiency syndrome, 209–239
Affect of client, 160
AIDS. *See* Acquired immunodeficiency syndrome
Anorexia, 72
Antisocial personality, 72
Anxiety, teaching theory and, 75–78
Arthritis, 155–158
As Good As It Gets, as teaching tool, 71
Autism, 73

Back Wards to Back Streets, as teaching tool, 69
A Beautiful Mind, as teaching tool, 69, 71
Behavioral Disorders in Children and Ordinary People, as teaching tool, 73
Beliefs, 160
Biomedical model, 1
    efficacy of, 1
    narrowness of, 1
Borderline antisocial personality, 72
Bulimia, 72

Care planning, 124–125
Care-provider attitude, 34
Caregiver concerns, 36–38
Caring, as objective of curriculum, 14, 17
Caring for Mo, as teaching tool, 73
Case examples, 147–158
Case models, 73

anxiety disorders, 71
biomedical, efficacy of, 1
chronic mental illness, 69
dissociative disorders, 72
eating disorders, 72
end of life, 73
mental disorders of childhood, adolescence, 73
mood disorders, 70
personality disorders, 72
psychotic disorders, 69
safety concerns, 71
substance-related disorders, 71
Chronic illness
    clinical skills, teaching, 87–132
    defined, 4
    educational environment, understanding, 9–20
    experience of students, 133–146
    living with, 1–7
    teaching stories, 21–41
    theory, teaching, 43–85
Chronic Illness: Impact and Interventions, as teaching tool, 29
Client teaching/learning project, guidelines for, 129
Client wellness interview, 166–168
    client description, 159
    summary, 159
    wellness, client perspective on, 159–165
Clinical component of teaching course design, 90–99

Clinical component of teaching
(*continued*)
course objectives, 88–90
medical-surgical component, 118–128
psychosocial-spiritual component, 99–118
student assessment, 128–131
Clinical evaluation tools, 185–194
completed, 195–207
Clinical judgment, essentials of, 28
Clinical Nursing: Pathophysiological & Psychosocial Approaches, as teaching tool, 1
Clinical objectives, 195
Cognition, client's, 161
Comfort zone, working outside of, 145–146
Community values, 13–14
Compassion, 12
Compliance issues, 31
Concept development, 16–17
Content emphasis, shift of, in teaching theory, 50
Content issues in teaching theory, 43–44, 48–50
Context
decisions reflecting, 121–122
importance of, 24–25
Coping with Chronic Illness: Overcoming Powerlessness, as teaching tool, 28–29
Courses in curriculum, 16
Critical thinking, 17, 194
as objective of curriculum, 14
Curriculum, 14–15
caring, concept of, 14, 17
client, focus on, 15, 16
concept development, 16–17
courses, 16
critical thinking, 14, 17
development of, 13
environment, 15, 16
health, 14, 16
nursing, 14–15
objectives of, 14–15

professional nursing, 15
professionalism, 17
program requirements, 15–17
program sequence, 16
values, 15–20
Customs of client, 160

Daily worksheet, 126
Deficit, language of, 27
Depression, 70
Development of curriculum, 13
Diabetes, 149–153
Dissociative disorders, 72
Documentation, 169–184
Dying to Be Thin, as teaching tool, 72

Eby-Booth, Ray, 11
Edgewood College
mission statement of, 10
overview of, 9–10
Educational environment, 9–20
Emphysema, 147–149
Empiric mode, narratives in, 54
End of life case model, 73
Environment, importance of, 15, 16, 190
Evaluation standards, 187–188
Evaluation tools, completed, 195–207
Experience of students, utilizing, 133–146

Faculty, 97–99
Family caregiving
challenges of, 36–37
extent of, 36–37
Fibromyalgia, 58–60
Fields, John, 10
Films, as teaching aids, 69–73
Final evaluation, 202–204
Flow of speech, client's, 160
flow of, 160
Focus of learning, 31–32
Foot care, 151
Foucault, Michel, 27
Future care, provision of, 123–124

Girl, Interrupted, as teaching tool, 72
Good Days, Bad Days, as teaching tool, 5, 50
Grace, moment of, 56–58
Gracefully Insane, as teaching tool, 50
Gray zone, nursing in, 23–24
Group participation, guidelines for, 169
Guidelines, independent experience, 116–118

Health, 16
derivation of word, 22
HIV. *See* Human immunodeficiency virus
Holistic perspective of, 22–25
Hospice, 142–144
Human immunodeficiency virus, 209–239
Hypertension, 153–155

Independent experience guidelines, 116–118
Individuality of style, 29–30
Insight of client, 161
Interview, wellness, 111–113, 159–168

Judgment, clinical, essentials of, 28
Judgment of client, 161
Justice, 11

Language, 44–46
Learning
organizing themes, 28–30
self-regulation theme, 30–33
Liver disease, 61–66
Logico-scientific mode, 25–28, 46
defined, 25
integration of, 25–28
Loss, understanding of, 136–144

Mania, 70
Medical-surgical nursing courses, 49, 118–128, 187–188
Medication sheet, 127
Medications management, 125–126

Mental illness, 66–78
Mentality of "us vs. them," impact of, 34
Midterm evaluation, 201–202
Miller, Judith, 28–29
Mission statement, Edgewood College, 10
Model
anxiety disorders, 71
biomedical, efficacy of, 1
chronic mental illness, 69
dissociative disorders, 72
eating disorders, 72
facing end of life, 73
mental disorders of childhood, adolescence, 73
mood disorders, 70
personality disorders, 72
psychotic disorders, 69
safety concerns, 71
substance-related disorders, 71
Mood of client, 160
Mr. Jones, as teaching tool, 70
Multiple substance abuse, 71

Narcissistic disorder, 72
Narrative mode, 25–28, 46
defined, 25
integration of, 25–28
strategy of, 26–28
National Council Licensure Exam, 47–48
NCLEX-RN. *See* National Council Licensure Exam
Noncompliance issues, 31
Nursing curriculum, 14–15
caring, 14, 17
client, 15, 16
concept development, 16–17
courses, 16
critical thinking, 14, 17
development of, 13
environment, 15, 16
health, 14, 16
objectives of, 14–15
professional nursing, 15

Nursing curriculum *(continued)*
  professionalism, 17
  program requirements, 15–17
  program sequence, 16
  values, 15–20
Nursing diagnosis, 2, 164–165
Nutrition, 173

Obesity, 72
Objectives of curriculum, 14–15
  caring, 14
  clients/person, 15
  critical thinking, 14
  environment, 15
  health, 14
  professional nursing, 15
Obsessive compulsive disorder, 71, 72
Organizing themes in learning, 28–30
Orientation, philosophical, 21
Outcome measures, 196–200

Partnership, 12–13
Pedagogy, 44–46
Philosophical orientation, 21
Physical fitness, 172–173
Positivist tradition of nursing, 23
Pregnancy, 139–142
Prince of Tides, as teaching tool, 72
Professional challenges, 136–139
Professional nursing, 15
Professionalism, 17
Program requirements, 15–17
Program sequence, 16
Progress note, wellness group, 175–177
Psychiatric nursing, 49
Psychosocial-spiritual component,
  99–118
  clinical evaluation tool, 195–207
  evaluation tools, 185
  methods, 108–118
  milieu, 99–101
  motives, 101–108

Quantum thinking, 22–23

Rate of speech, client's, flow of, 160
Rehabilitation, client response, 34

Relationships/intimacy, 174
Religious affiliation, 160
Remen, Rachel, 20
Restraints, 71
Role of teacher, 133–136

Sample wellness group plan, 169–170
  group format, structure, 170
  group participation, guidelines for,
    169
  member criteria, 169
  nutrition, 173
  orientation, 170–172
  physical fitness, 172–173
  purpose, statement of, 169
  rationale, 169
  relationships/intimacy, 174
  session overviews, 170
    orientation, 170–172
  spirituality, 174
  stress management, 172
  target population, description of,
    169
Sample wellness group progress note,
  175–177
Sample wellness interview, 159–168
Schizophrenia, 69
Seclusion, impact of, 71
Self-regulation theme, 30–33, 49
Sensorium, of client, 161
Site selection, 91–97
Speech of client, 160
Speech patterns, 160
Spiritual orientation, 99–118, 160, 174
Stigma, 33–36, 49
  derivation of word, 34–35
  social construction of, 69
Stories, in teaching, 21–41
  care-provider attitude, 34
  caregiver concerns, 36–38
  clinical judgment, essentials of, 28
  compliance, 31
  context, importance of, 24–25
  deficit, language of, 27
  family caregiving

challenges of, 36–37
  extent of, 36–37
focus of learning, 31–32
gray zone, nursing in, 23–24
health, derivation of word, 22
holistic perspective of, 22–25
individuality of style, 29–30
learning
  organizing themes, 28–30
  self-regulation theme, 30–33
logico-scientific mode, 25–28
  defined, 25
  integration of, 25–28
mentality of "us vs.them," impact of, 34
narrative mode
  defined, 25
  strategy of, 26–28
narrative modes, 25–28
  integration of, 25–28
noncompliance, 31
philosophical orientation, 21
positivist tradition of nursing, 23
quantum thinking, 22–23
rehabilitation, client response, 34
self-regulation, conceptualization of, 30–32
stigma, 33–36
  derivation of word, 34–35
treatment, client response, 34
vocabulary, power of, 26–27
whole-person care, 22–25
worldview, effect of, 32–33
Stress management, 172
Substance abuse, 71

Target population, description of, 169
Teaching, use of stories, 21–41
Teaching project, 126–128, 129
Teaching theory, 43–85
  ability to practice, 47
  and tests, 47
  anxiety, 75–78
  case studies, 60–66
  content, 48–50, 49
  content emphasis, shift of, 50

content issues, 43–44
course objectives, 43–44
empiric mode, narratives in, 54
end of life case model, 73
fibromyalgia, 58–60
films, as teaching aids, 69–73
grace, moment of, 56–58
impromptu stories, 75–78
language, 44–46
liver disease, 61–66
logico-scientific mode, 46
medical-surgical nursing courses, 49
mental illness, 66–78
narrative modes, 46
pedagogy, paradoxical, 44–46
process, 50–54
psychiatric nursing, 49
self-regulation, 49
setting tone stories, 54–58
stigma, 49
student assessment, 46–48
student stories, 58–60
tests, 47
texts, election of, 48–49
Tests, 47
Texts, election of, 48–49
Traditions, customs, 160
Treatment, client response, 34
Truth, 10–11
Tuesdays With Morrie, as teaching tool, 50
28 Days, as teaching tool, 71

Values, 10–14, 15–20
  community, 13–14
  compassion, 12
  justice, 11
  partnership, 12–13
  truth, 10–11
Videos, 69–73
Vocabulary, power of, 26–27

Wellness group
  documentation, 169–184
  progress note, 175–177
  sample plan, 169–170

Wellness interviews, 111–113, 159–168   Worksheet, use of, 126
Whole-person care, 22–25   Worldview, effect of, 32–33
Wit, as teaching tool, 73